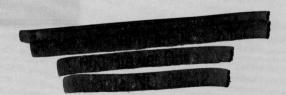
The Medical Examiner

by Toney Allman

LUCENT BOOKS

An imprint of Thomson Gale, a part of The Thomson Corporation

THOMSON

★

GALE
™

Detroit • New York • San Francisco • San Diego • New Haven, Conn. • Waterville, Maine • London • Munich

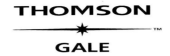

Acknowledgement

We would like to express our sincere gratitude to Dr. Christina Stanley, Chief Deputy Medical Examiner of the San Diego County Medical Examiner's Office, for her invaluable reviews of Lucent's Crime Scene Investigations: *The Medical Examiner.*

For more information, contact
Lucent Books
27500 Drake Rd.
Farmington Hills, MI 48331-3535
Or you can visit our Internet site at http://www.gale.com

LIBRARY OF CONGRESS CATALOGING-IN-PUBLICATION DATA

Allman, Toney.
  The medical examiner / by Toney Allman.
    p. cm. — (Crime scene investigations series)
  Includes bibliographical references and index.
  ISBN 1-59018-912-4 (hard cover : alk. paper)
    1. Forensic pathology—Juvenile literature. 2. Medical examiners
(Law)—Juvenile literature.   I. Title. II. Series.
  RA1063.4.A47 2006
  614'.1—dc22

                    2005025371

Contents

Foreword

The popularity of crime scene and investigative crime shows on television has come as a surprise to many who work in the field. The main surprise is the concept that crime scene analysts are the true crime solvers, when in truth, it takes dozens of people, doing many different jobs, to solve a crime. Often, the crime scene analyst's contribution is a small one. One Minnesota forensic scientist says that the public "has gotten the wrong idea. Because I work in a lab similar to the ones on *CSI*, people seem to think I'm solving crimes left and right—just me and my microscope. They don't believe me when I tell them that it's the investigators that are solving crimes, not me."

Crime scene analysts do have an important role to play, however. Science has rapidly added a whole new dimension to gathering and assessing evidence. Modern crime labs can match a hair of a murder suspect to one found on a murder victim, for example, or recover a latent fingerprint from a threatening letter, or use a powerful microscope to match tool marks made during the wiring of an explosive device to a tool in a suspect's possession.

Probably the most exciting of the forensic scientist's tools is DNA analysis. DNA can be found in just one drop of blood, a dribble of saliva on a toothbrush, or even the residue from a fingerprint. Some DNA analysis techniques enable scientists to tell with certainty, for example, whether a drop of blood on a suspect's shirt is that of a murder victim.

While these exciting techniques are now an essential part of many investigations, they cannot solve crimes alone. "DNA doesn't come with a name and address on it," says the Minnesota forensic scientist. "It's great if you have someone in custody to match the sample to, but otherwise, it doesn't help. That's the investigator's job. We can have all the great DNA evidence in the world, and without a suspect, it will just sit on the shelf. We've all seen cases with very little forensic evidence get solved by the resourcefulness of a detective."

While forensic specialists get the most media attention today, the work of detectives still forms the core of most criminal investigations. Their job, in many ways, has changed little over the years. Most cases are still solved through the persistence and determination of a criminal detective whose work may be anything but glamorous. Many cases require routine, even mind-numbing tasks. After the July 2005 bombings in London, for example, police officers sat in front of video players watching thousands of hours of closed-circuit television tape from security cameras throughout the city, and as a result were able to get the first images of the bombers.

The Lucent Books Crime Scene Investigations series explores the variety of ways crimes are solved. Titles cover particular crimes such as murder, specific cases such as the killing of three civil rights workers in Mississippi, or the role specialists such as medical examiners play in solving crimes. Each title in the series demonstrates the ways a crime may be solved, from the various applications of forensic science and technology to the reasoning of investigators. Sidebars examine both the limits and possibilities of the new technologies and present crime statistics, career information, and step-by-step explanations of scientific and legal processes.

The Crime Scene Investigations series strives to be both informative and realistic about how members of law enforcement—criminal investigators, forensic scientists, and others—solve crimes, for it is essential that student researchers understand that crime solving is rarely quick or easy. Many factors—from a detective's dogged pursuit of one tenuous lead to a suspect's careless mistakes to sheer luck to complex calculations computed in the lab—are all part of crime solving today.

Death Detectives

When Thomas T. Noguchi first joined the Los Angeles County Coroner's Office in 1960, he found himself in cramped rooms in the basement of the Hall of Justice. Until the middle of the 1980s many other medical examiners throughout the United States were in similar circumstances. They worked in the dingy basements of hospitals or city morgues or even at funeral homes. One medical examiner in New York once performed an autopsy in the middle of a field, just to make the point that medical examiners received little respect and were rarely acknowledged for their ability to solve crimes. Today, however, more and more medical examiners occupy modern forensic centers and have the very latest technology and equipment at their disposal. Forensic medical examiners have become indispensable members of crime-solving teams throughout the country. They use their medical expertise and their skill in criminal investigation to function as death detectives.

Forensics is the use of scientific technology to investigate crimes and discover evidence that will be used in a court of law. Pathology is the medical investigation of the causes of diseases and deaths. A forensic pathologist combines both occupations. He or she is a medical doctor who specializes in criminal investigations, especially as medicine applies to violent death or murder. In some parts of the country forensic pathologists are called coroners. Others are known as medical examiners, or MEs, for short. Whatever their title, forensic pathologists help the living by discovering the truth about death. Noguchi, who went on to become the chief medical examiner of Los Angeles County, once said, "In every death, there is a mystery until the cause is known. Was it natural or unnatural, a

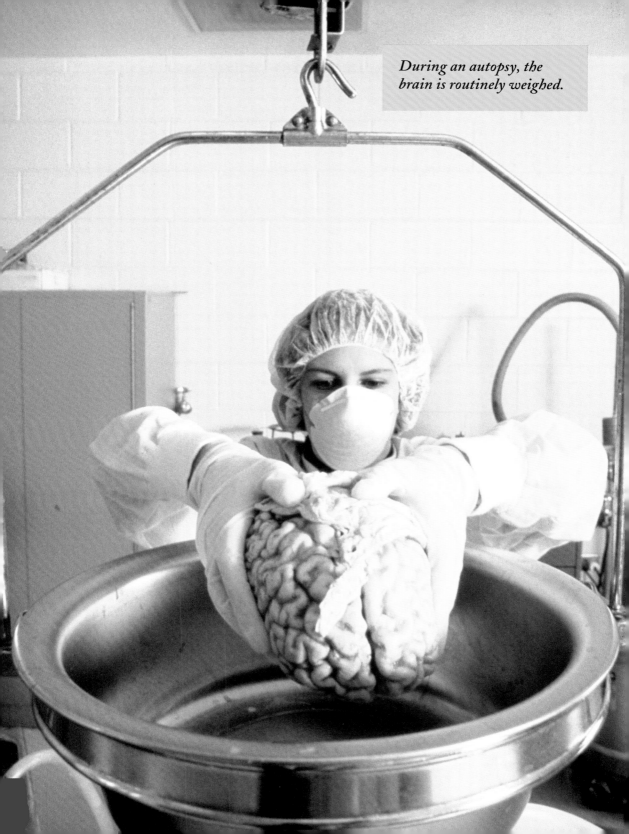

During an autopsy, the brain is routinely weighed.

homicide, a suicide, or an accident? A coroner is, if you will, a medical detective who is specifically trained to solve that mystery." He adds, "In every death there are lessons to be learned for the living."[1]

Noguchi's "lessons to be learned" include finding who is guilty of murder and who is not. He and other medical examiners are often responsible for pointing the way to capturing and convicting perpetrators of crimes. Sometimes MEs exonerate the innocent as well, by proving that deaths were not homicides but accidents or suicides, or by demonstrating that medical evidence points to an unsuspected individual in a murder. Medical examiners accomplish these feats in modern facilities with high-powered equipment and a staff of specialists that were unheard of just a few decades ago. A tour of today's forensic laboratory reveals an amazing combination of science, medicine, and forensic investigative tools that are part of the medical examiner's arsenal.

Medical examiners today perform autopsies in modern, well-equipped laboratories like this one.

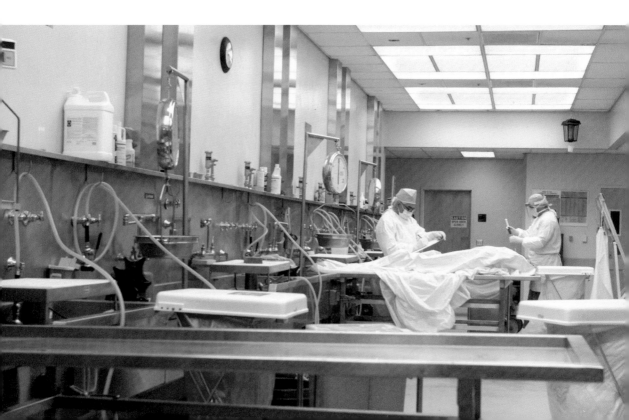

The Los Angeles County Forensic Science Center, for example, which is representative of others in major cities around the country, is set up for the complete and total investigation of suspicious, unexplained, or unexpected death. With autopsy rooms, specialized laboratories, and evidence rooms, the facility is devoted to the many different aspects of work that may be necessary to solve the mystery of death.

In the United States today, most medical examiners work out of large cities, although their responsibility may extend to large areas of a state. Fewer than five hundred trained forensic pathologists currently practice as medical examiners, and their skills are in high demand. In about half of jurisdictions across the country other doctors or regular pathologists from hospitals perform the work of medical examiners for their cities or counties. Some towns have no medical examiner at all, just a person who acts as a coroner and collects dead bodies when the police are through with them. As a result, forensic pathologists are often asked to review cases and use their expertise to help in homicide investigations across the country. Without the contributions of forensic pathologists who act as medical examiners, many murders would go unsolved.

Michael Bader, a renowned New York forensic pathologist, has consulted on homicide cases throughout the country.

CHAPTER 1

At the Death Scene

A phone call awoke Frederick Zugibe the night of April 22, 1973. He was chief medical examiner of Rockland County, New York, and the call was a request for his services. The body of a little girl had been discovered in a state park. Police suspected that it was seven-year-old Joan D'Alessandro, who had disappeared from her neighborhood three days before. Zugibe arrived at the park in about an hour and discovered police, detectives, photographers, reporters, and concerned citizens tramping about the scene. "I want every unauthorized person out of this area now!"[2] he yelled at the top of his voice. Zugibe was protecting the integrity of the crime scene, as was his right and responsibility. He was beginning his attempt to determine the story Joan's body had to tell by establishing the cause, manner, and mechanism, or circumstances, of the death.

Starting the Story

A medical examiner is charged with discovering the cause, manner, and mechanism of death when a death is sudden, unexpected, or suspicious. The cause of death is the injury or disease that leads to the death. It may be a bullet wound, a stabbing, poison, blunt trauma, or any number of violent actions, as well as natural causes such as diseases. The mechanism of death may be shock, blood loss, cardiac arrest, or any of the other ways that a person dies in response to an injury or disease. There are five possible manners of death: homicide, suicide, accident, natural, or unknown. The last is reserved for those cases in which the medical examiner cannot determine with certainty the manner in which a person died.

Where there is a death, medical examiners isolate the crime scene to preserve evidence.

Neither Zugibe nor anyone else questioned the manner in which Joan D'Alessandro died. It was clearly homicide. Zugibe's investigation into the cause and manner of Joan's death began immediately. Since part of any homicide story involves who did it, he also sought to discover clues that would lead to her killer. Zugibe once explained, "The more accurate this story proves to be, experience tells, the faster the investigation will proceed, and the more apt we will be to track down the bad guy."[3] In their official capacity, all MEs or their staff supervise the collection of death scene evidence, interview witnesses, evaluate the circumstances in the environment, and examine the body as the first steps in fulfilling their responsibility. Rarely does the crime scene answer all the medical examin-

Specially trained police officers take fingerprints from bodies as an aid to identification.

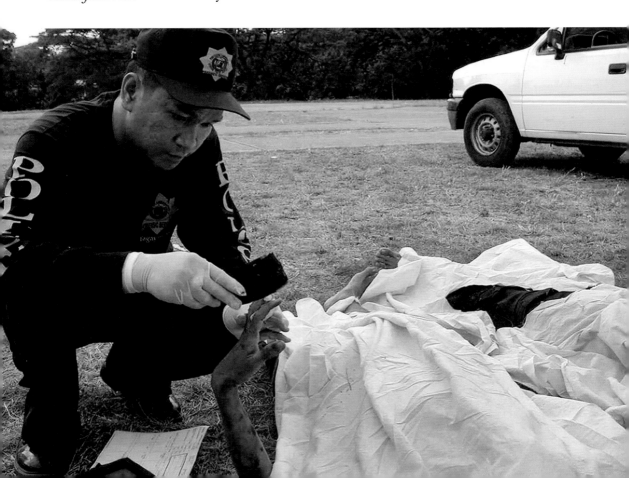

er's questions, but usually the place where a body is found yields valuable clues about the cause, manner, and mechanism of death. In this case, however, the environment where Joan was found had been contaminated by all the people present. Still, the body itself remained undisturbed. Joan's body was where Zugibe began his investigation.

Zugibe squatted down to examine the body and to look for clues. The cause of death was obvious. The body lay on its back, wedged between two large rocks. The girl's neck was twisted unnaturally to one side, and she was nude, with many cuts and bruises covering her skin. Zugibe's initial estimate of the cause of death was that Joan had been beaten and strangled. Because she was nude and her clothing was found folded in a nearby plastic bag, he assumed that she had also been sexually molested.

Rigor, Livor, and Algor Mortis

Immediately he discovered evidence that would help him establish the time of death and perhaps lead to a suspect. Time of death can be difficult to establish, but clues in the body can help. Zugibe tried to estimate time of death by checking for stiffness of the body (rigor mortis), measuring body temperature (algor mortis), and looking for pooling of blood in body tissues (livor mortis).

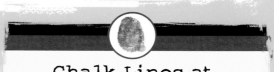

Chalk Lines at Crime Scenes

Movies and television programs often show investigators drawing a chalk outline around a dead body. In truth, however, at crime scenes today, a body is extensively photographed, carefully examined for evidence, and eventually moved by a qualified death investigator. No outlines of where the body lay are needed once the investigation is complete. Therefore, the police and the medical examiner have no need to draw chalk lines around a dead body.

Some people think that the first person to popularize chalk lines was the film director Alfred Hitchcock, who probably showed murder scenes with chalk tracings of the victim for dramatic effect. In the decades since Hitchcock's movies were made, movie and television studios have continued the practice, but it is not a reflection of current real life crime scene investigations.

Causes of Death in the United States

93% of deaths are due to natural causes (old age and disease)

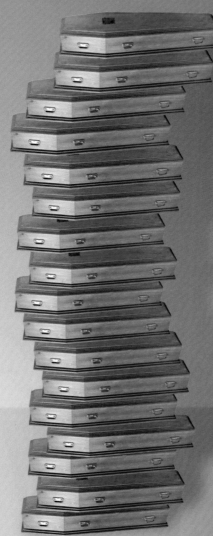

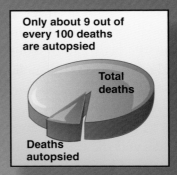

Only about 9 out of every 100 deaths are autopsied

Total deaths

Deaths autopsied

7% of deaths are due to unnatural causes (accidental, suicide, homicide, and undetermined)

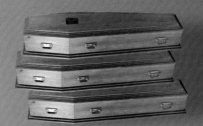

Source: *American Demographic*, April 1997.

After a person stops breathing, the body's muscle cells no longer receive oxygen and begin to stiffen. Rigor mortis can first be noticed in the small muscles in the face and then spreads throughout the large muscles of the body. About twelve hours after death all the muscles are so rigid that joints will not bend. Then rigor mortis slowly disappears, starting at the bottom of the body and moving upward. After about thirty-six hours rigor mortis is gone, and the body is flexible again. This process, however, can be faster or slower depending on such things as air temperature and even body weight. Bodies enter rigor mortis faster in hot environments than cold ones. Small bodies go through rigor mortis more quickly than large ones. Zugibe noted that Joan's body was completely out of rigor mortis; therefore she had been dead at least thirty-six hours.

An Important Clue

Algor mortis refers to the decrease in body temperature after death. Adult bodies cool at a rate of about 1.5 degrees per hour until they take on the temperature of the surrounding air. Zugibe measured the air temperature where Joan's body was found and also took the temperature of the body. The temperatures were the same, which also suggested that she had been dead for at least thirty-six hours.

The most important clue Zugibe discovered was the livor mortis, or discoloration, on Joan's body. Livor mortis occurs when blood pools in the body after the heart stops pumping. Blood collects in particular body areas because of gravity. A body that lies face down, for example, will show dark discolorations on the chest and stomach. A body on its back has blood pooled in the buttocks and back. After about six to eight hours this blood is fixed in place even if the body is moved. Before that time, blood will slowly flow with gravity if a body is put into a new position.

The darkened areas on Joan's skin were fixed, but that did not help much with determining the time of death. Zugibe already knew that she had been dead more than eight hours.

However, livor mortis provided him with an important piece of evidence. Joan was lying on her back, but the livor mortis was on her stomach. Zugibe said, "So we already know that Joan was murdered in another location, left in that spot for more than six hours while the blood settled and congealed, then dumped here in Rockland."[4] It was impossible for livor mortis to have been on Joan's stomach unless she had lain on her stomach for several hours after death. This critical piece of information was eventually part of the accumulation of evidence that led to the capture of Joan's killer. He had killed her in his house, left the body in his basement until nightfall, and then driven to the park and dumped the body far away from his home.

Poking into Everything

Despite the initially contaminated crime scene, Joan's killer was caught, but often a disturbed scene thwarts justice. Zugibe

Homicide investigators survey the crime scene and take photographs before a body is moved.

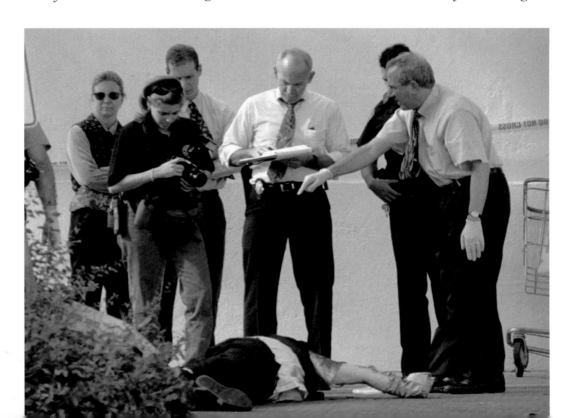

knew this when he ordered everyone away that April night. His responsibility was to examine the whole scene as a medical detective. Crime scenes must be protected until the medical examiner or a representative arrives and takes control. Michael M. Baden, a New York medical examiner, says, "It is the job of the first police officer on the scene to set up a perimeter through which only the necessary homicide detectives, laboratory personnel and medical examiners should be allowed to pass." He adds, "The first hour of a scene is critical and . . . in those sixty minutes the evidence can either be protected or destroyed. It all depends on the perimeter established."[5]

Within the perimeter of an undisturbed crime scene, the medical examiner oversees a search for evidence as obvious as a pool of blood or as insignificant as a single hair. The search for minute, or trace, evidence is based on Locard's Exchange Principle, which states that no one can enter a space without leaving some sign, however small, of having been there. Baden says,

By the Numbers

16,137

Number of murders in the United States in 2004

> When you walk into a room, you change it. In fact, how you enter and exit changes things. Enter, turn around and walk right out, touching nothing, and you have still left something of yourself behind—a grain of sand from the sole of your shoe, perhaps, or a fiber from the carpet of your car. It could be a hair—yours or that of someone you touched earlier.
>
> Enter a room and have a physical fight with someone and you will change that room, yourself, and the other person by what you exchange. It's very simple: When

any two objects come into contact with each other, there is always a transfer from one object to another.[6]

In addition to trace evidence, other evidence may provide clues that help tell the story of a death. Baden explains, "Virtually anything could be a clue—fibers, bullets, chewing gum on a shirt, a cigarette butt on the heel of a shoe, flecks of paint, garden soil, or sand beneath a fingernail." When bodies are found indoors, he says, "at the scene we poke around, looking at empty whiskey bottles, what is on the stove or in the fridge, whether there is digitalis or insulin in the medicine chest, sleeping pills or Prozac, cocaine or heroin."[7]

Follow Your Nose

A medical examiner's investigation includes a search for any relevant information, anywhere. In his work as a medical examiner in Los Angeles, Thomas Noguchi always began his crime scene investigations by looking at the ceiling. He says, "Don't worry about the body; the body will stay there. . . . First examine the room in a systematic, preplanned way, beginning with the ceiling. Clues may be up there: bullet holes, bloodstains, chipped plaster."[8] From the ceiling, his attention then moved to the walls and furniture, searching for any important pieces of information. Investigators collect hairs and blood spots, for example, so that the medical examiner's office can test them to determine the manner of death and perhaps help identify suspects in homicides. Any such clues may also help the medical examiner to establish the means of death.

Noguchi's careful examination of one crime scene led to the discovery that it was in fact a crime scene. Along with detectives from the Los Angeles Police Department, he was called to an empty house where an abandoned dog was barking and blood stained the walls of the bathroom. The only clue that Noguchi found was an odd smell and a yellow stain in the bathtub. Because of his medical training, Noguchi recognized the smell as sulfuric acid, a highly corrosive chemical. He recalls,

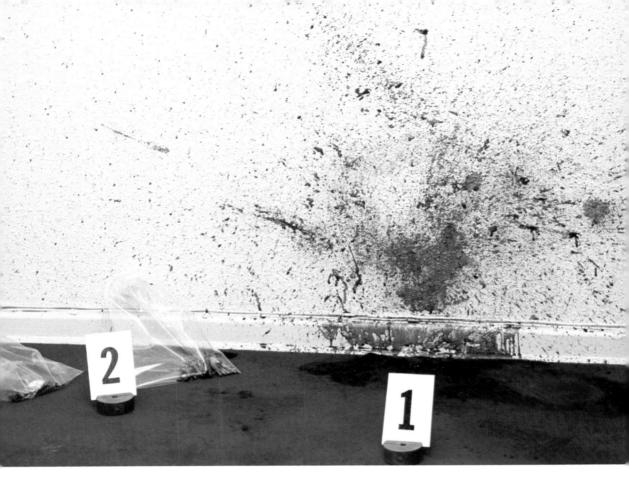

"And at that moment, I felt a little chill of horror as I realized the possible significance of the smell coupled with that stain. I ordered the whole bathroom dug up." Once the tub was removed and the pipes under the house revealed, Noguchi climbed into the workmen's hole and examined the drain trap that led to the sewer system. He found tiny pieces of evidence caught in the trap—two human teeth. Noguchi realized what the teeth meant: "A human body had been dissolved in acid in the tub and then washed down the drain."[9] Once police knew to look for a suspect who had access to sulfuric acid, they quickly identified one of the men who had lived in that house. He worked at a factory where sulfuric acid was used. He had killed his roommate in a fight and then disposed of the body down the bathtub drain. Thanks to Noguchi's careful on-scene investigation, the murderer was brought to justice.

Evidence that cannot be moved, such as spatters and pools of blood, are marked and photographed, while items that can be moved are placed in bags.

Use Your Head

Seemingly insignificant clues have helped identify many a murderer. Zugibe once helped solve a case by looking at trees. He had been called to an outdoor murder scene where the body of victim Susan Reeve had been found. He remembers, "In examining Reeve's naked body, I notice a number of long, pointed yellow leaves embedded in the upper parts of her chest and abdomen." These leaves were stuck into the dead woman's skin, telling Zugibe that she must have been lying face down for a number of hours after death. He knew the leaves were from a weeping willow tree, so he looked around at the crime scene in curiosity. "I walk around the immediate area and look for their source, but there are no weeping willow trees to be found," he says. "None within several

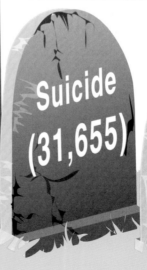

Causes of Unnatural Deaths in the United States

Accidental (106,742)

Suicide (31,655)

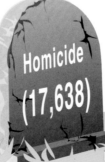

Homicide (17,638)

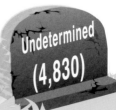

Undetermined (4,830)

hundred feet of the body; none within several hundred yards."[10] His inspection of the crime scene and the discovery of the leaves proved that Reeve had been killed elsewhere. The police were able to identify that place and eventually catch the murderer.

A Medical Examiner's Investigator

In some parts of the country the medical examiner does not visit the crime scene personally but sends a trained death investigator to secure the body and begin the investigation. Mary Fran Ernst is a forensic nurse and a death investigator for the St. Louis Medical Examiner's office in Missouri. As the medical examiner's representative, she once found evidence that a supposed homicide was really an accident. Police called her to a garage in which five bodies had been found. When she arrived at the scene Ernst first noted that the garage doors had been shut up tightly, and the area was very hot. A gun lay beside one of the victims. Police assumed that all five victims had been shot in a mass murder, but Ernst crouched down and systematically examined the bodies. She found no signs of any gunshot wounds or other injuries.

Then Ernst noticed the fingernails of each victim. The bases of the nails were a cherry red color. Ernst knew from her medical training that red nail beds were a sign of carbon monoxide poisoning. She directed the police investigation to a car in the garage. They found evidence that the car had been left running. It had finally run out of gas or stalled, but too late. The car's carbon monoxide exhaust—odorless and colorless—had overwhelmed the victims before they knew what was happening. With no fresh air in the tightly shut garage, the car's exhaust had acted like a poison. Unaware, the victims had breathed the carbon monoxide, lost consciousness, and died in a tragic accident. Ernst had discovered the cause, manner, and mechanism of death right at the crime scene and was able to make an accurate report to the medical examiner. She remarked, "Dead people do talk to you; you just have to listen really carefully. Their bodies tell us what happened."[11]

Becoming a Forensic Nurse

Job Description:
In medical examiner offices, forensic nurses are commonly charged with documenting and investigating death, attempting to determine cause and manner of death, and assisting the medical examiner however necessary. A forensic nurse may work in a medical examiner's office, operate in a hospital intake setting, or help an elected county coroner by functioning as a medical expert.

Education:
A forensic nurse first has to have a degree as a registered nurse. He or she then attends a school program to get an advanced degree or certificate in forensic nursing.

Qualifications:
To be certified, the forensic nurse must pass the Certified Forensic Nurse examination sponsored by the American College of Forensic Examiners and be certified by the International Association of Forensic Nurses and/or the American Board of Medicolegal Death Investigators.

Additional Information:
A forensic nurse needs to possess the skills and knowledge to conduct an on-scene death investigation, have a working knowledge of the laws of his or her jurisdiction, and possess excellent verbal and written communication skills. Forensic nurses must be able to conduct meaningful eyewitness or family interviews, relate to grieving survivors and family members, and interview and counsel rape or other crime victims.

Salary:
$35,000–$60,000

Documenting Death

Determinations of the means and manner of death are extremely important parts of the medical examiner's story, but in homicides the crime investigation cannot stop there. A critical part of the investigation is documenting the site. Photographs are taken of the crime scene. The body itself is carefully photographed, with close-ups from many different angles. Only afterward is the body moved, perhaps turned over, and searched for more clues. If important evidence is discovered, such as knife or bullet wounds, they are also photographed. Any trace evidence under the body is carefully collected, too.

Another responsibility of the medical examiner is to formally declare the victim dead and later, to issue a death certificate. Only a medical doctor can say for sure that a person is

Investigators photograph the body and its surroundings before it is moved.

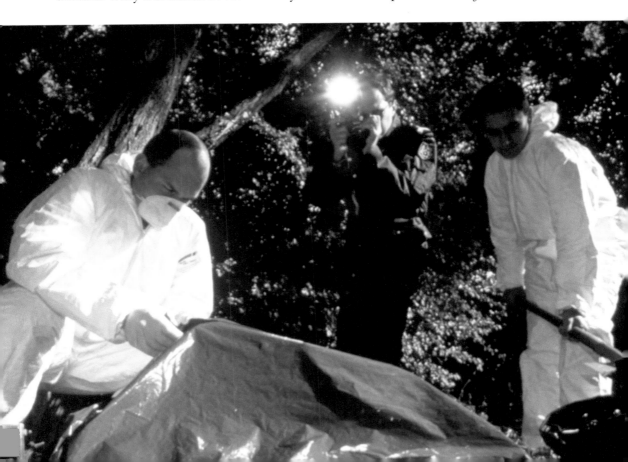

dead. On rare occasions, persons who have been presumed dead were not. This can happen, for instance, from severe electric shocks or occasionally from drowning. Under these circumstances, Zugibe explains, "All the classic sights and sounds of life cease; but deep inside the beat goes on, undetectable by all but the most sensitive medical instruments."[12] Even in cases like Joan's, where death is obvious, by law the medical examiner makes the formal declaration of death.

Removing the Body

Finally, the medical examiner or his or her deputy supervises the removal of the body, taking great care not to disturb any evidence that may exist on the body. The body, Baden says, "in itself, is a crime scene." An identifying tag is placed

Only after all evidence has been gathered and documented is a body removed from the crime scene.

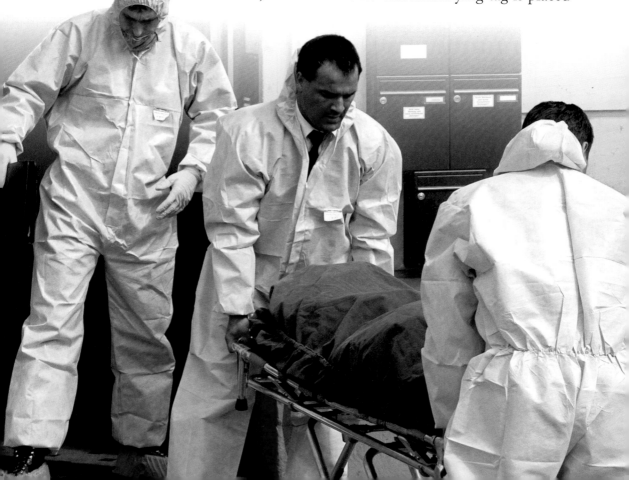

on a convenient spot on the body, usually on a toe or a foot. The tag establishes a "chain of evidence"[13] that records each person who handles the body. It also ensures that a body will not get mixed up with another at the end of its trip. Then the hands and feet of the victim are carefully placed in balloonlike bags that are tied at the wrists and the ankles. These bags trap any evidence that may be on hands and feet so that clues will not be lost.

After the bags are in place the body is wrapped in a white sheet that investigators bring to the scene. White sheets are used because specks of evidence are easier to see on white than on another color. A sheet from the victim's own home, however, must never be used since it would contaminate any trace evidence on the body. Baden explains, "With a clean sheet brought to the scene, anything that falls on it will have come from the victim and perhaps whomever he came in contact with during those last moments of his life."[14]

The body in its wrapping is placed in a body bag. Body bags are made of tough, flexible fabric that can protect the contents should they be, for example, dragged along a forest floor or hoisted into a helicopter. The bag is zipped up, and the body is finally ready for transport. Now the most important work of the medical examiner truly begins.

CHAPTER 2

Autopsy

An autopsy is a specialized medical procedure that supplies critical information in a death investigation. Missouri medical examiner Jay Dix says, "A forensic pathologist must determine how and why a person died by performing a thorough autopsy and studying the results of a good scene investigation. Both are essential in determining the correct cause, manner, and mechanism of death." He adds, "Cause of death is the most important piece of information obtained from an autopsy."[15] During an autopsy the medical examiner inspects and dissects a corpse to make it tell the story of its death.

In the Morgue

Most bodies are stored in refrigerated units until the medical examiner can do the autopsy. These units are kept at about 38°F (3.3°C), cold enough to preserve the body but not cold enough to freeze and damage tissues. When the ME is ready, the body is brought into the autopsy room.

Autopsy rooms are well lighted but usually windowless. They are equipped with air conditioning, but MEs often turn it off, so that no stray breeze can blow away any evidence. The autopsy table is often two-tiered. The top tier, where the body lies, is perforated so that blood and other fluids can run down to the collection tray below and not be lost. Beside the table lie all the instruments that will be used during the autopsy. Baden once remarked, "There you see scalpels. Here, lying next to the scalpels, are a bread knife, pruning clippers and a vibrating bone saw."[16] In addition, most MEs use scissors, a magnifying glass, ultraviolet lights, X-ray machines, and a series of collection bottles and envelopes for holding tissue samples and

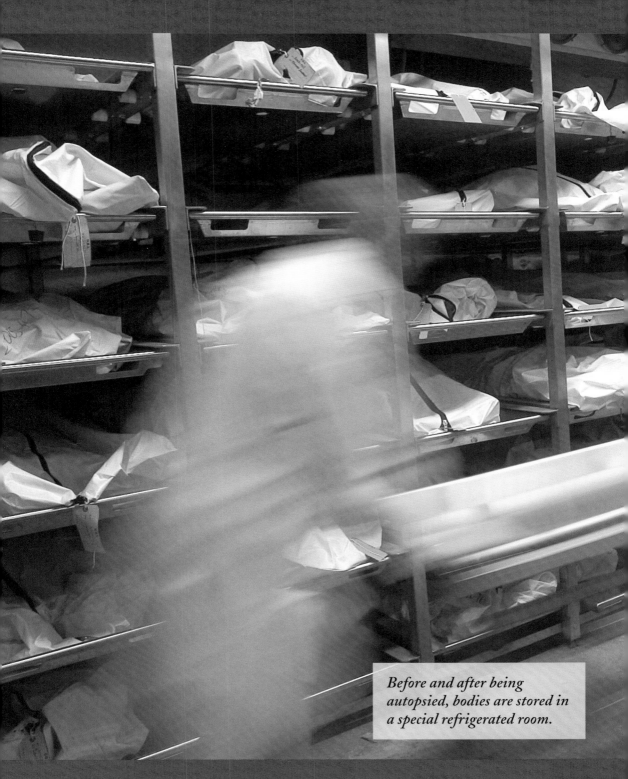

Before and after being autopsied, bodies are stored in a special refrigerated room.

trace evidence. Before beginning the autopsy the medical examiner dresses in a hospital gown or surgical scrubs, an apron, mask, and goggles or other eye protection. Booties, gloves, and a hair cap are added to prevent contamination of trace evidence on the body.

A medical examiner takes samples from under a victim's fingernails in search of skin, hair, or fibers from the killer.

External Examination

An external examination of the body is the medical examiner's first step. The body is removed from the body bag and laid face up on the table. Before the body bag is discarded, however, it is examined for evidence. Says Baden, "If the body was wrapped properly, there should be little information in the bag—it should be inside the sheet and on the body. But you always check."[17] Then the sheet is unwrapped and also inspected.

Once the body is revealed, it is photographed, and the clothes are inspected for tears, bullet holes, or trace evidence such as fibers or blood. Then the clothing is removed. The hand and foot bags are removed and inspected, too. Any trace evidence is placed in small envelopes and saved. Fingernails are examined, and scrapings from under the nails are taken, since blood, skin, or fibers from the murderer may be under a victim's fingernails.

Next the medical examiner does a detailed visual examination of the body, first with the naked eye and then with a magnifying glass. Even if an obvious injury is present, the ME does not assume it caused the death. Methodically, the ME examines the body from head to foot, noting any wounds, scrapes, or bruises. Every wound is photographed and measured. Every body part has the potential of yielding a clue to the story of the death.

Tiny hemorrhages like this one on the eyelids may indicate that the victim was suffocated.

Eyes, for instance, are examined for tiny pinpoint blood spots known as petechial hemorrhages. Such hemorrhages might indicate that a death was not natural but caused by suffocation or strangulation. They occur because the victim's veins swell and tiny capillaries break when the blood cannot return to the heart.

Enid Gilbert, a pediatric pathologist in Wisconsin, once used the presence of petechial hemorrhages to prove that Sandra Pankow, a babysitter, was a serial killer. Three babies had died in Pankow's home. The original hospital diagnosis for each of the children's deaths had been that it was a tragic but natural death—Sudden Infant Death Syndrome, or SIDS. Pathologists, however, were suspicious. Medical examiner Vincent Di Maio insisted, "Two SIDS deaths [in the same family or nursery] is improbable. But three is impossible."[18] The babies' bodies were exhumed, or dug up from their graves, and Gilbert did the autopsies. Along with other evidence she found petechial hemorrhages in the eyes of one child. Babies who die of SIDS, which has no known cause, never have such hemorrhages. Pankow was tried and convicted of smothering the children.

Minute Clues

Careful body examination may also reveal needle marks on the skin from drug injection. These marks might indicate a drug user who overdosed accidentally, but they may also point to an unsuspected homicide. A medical examiner in England, David Price, discovered such a murder. A nurse, Kenneth Barlow, reported that he had found his wife drowned in the bathtub. Price, however, after careful examination discovered two tiny needle marks on the dead woman's buttocks. Barlow had given his wife insulin shots, which lowered her blood sugar so much that she passed out. Then he had put her in the bathtub to drown. Thanks to Price's magnifying glass, Barlow was convicted of murder.

Choking and Cutting

Most autopsies do not depend on discovering clues as small as needle marks. Usually, murder is dramatically apparent. Zugibe says, "If a particularly violent crime is committed, the corpse can be disfigured in ways that most people who have never visited a torture chamber can scarcely imagine."[19] The medical examiner often sees the cause of death by looking at visible wounds. Strangulations, for example, are evident in bruises on the neck. The body of Joan D'Alessandro showed these wounds. When a cord or wire is used to strangle a victim, it can leave an obvious mark. Says Dix, "If a ligature [a constricting device] is thin like a rope, a depressed mark on the neck is usually apparent and the pattern can be matched to a particular ligature."[20]

Stab wounds are as visible as ligature marks. Medical examiners measure the width and depth of each stab wound. Often the size and type of blade can be estimated by the size

Inside the Autopsy Room

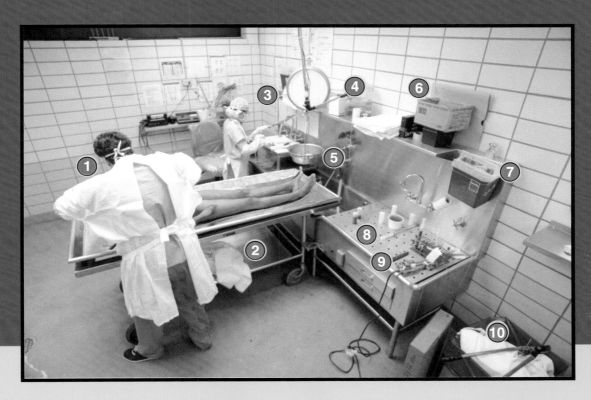

1. The ME and assistants wear protective clothing for hygiene and to avoid contaminating the evidence.

2. The body is dissected on a stainless-steel table, tilted so body fluids drain at one end.

3. The ME closely examines the body's internal organs in this area.

4. A microphone suspended from the ceiling lets the ME record observations during the autopsy.

5. A hanging scale is used for weighing organs.

6. This box is for storing X-rays.

7. This box, called a "sharps container," is for disposal of needles and scalpel blades.

8. Tissue samples, blood, and stomach contents are placed in containers for analysis in the lab.

9. An electric vibrating saw is used for cutting the skull bones.

10. This tool is used for cutting the rib cage.

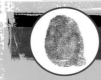

Becoming a Forensic Pathologist

Job Description:
As a certified forensic pathologist, the medical examiner oversees and performs autopsies, is responsible for death investigations as they relate to the evidence on and within the body, and writes autopsy reports that describe as completely as possible the cause, mechanism, and manner of death. The forensic pathologist has jurisdiction over any death suspected of being unnatural—violent or accidental, any unexplained death, unclaimed bodies, contaminated bodies, and infants suspected of dying of SIDS.

Education:
After finishing college, the aspiring forensic pathologist must complete four years of medical school. Next the new doctor undergoes a residency program in pathology for an additional three to five years. The pathologist then trains in the subspecialty of forensics at a fellowship training program that lasts one to two years. These studies include toxicology (the study of toxins), criminalistics (the use of science in criminal investigations), radiology (imaging technology such as X-rays), ballistics (bullets), serology (blood), and other medical-legal sciences.

Qualifications:
Once his or her education is completed, the forensic pathologist achieves board certification through examination by the National Association of Medical Examiners.

Additional Information:
A certified forensic pathologist must have good communication skills, be able to write clear autopsy reports, and be prepared to testify to autopsy findings in court. A chief medical examiner is also responsible for overseeing the work of other medical examiners as well as the forensics science laboratories under his office's jurisdiction.

Salary:
$60,000–$200,000

and shape of the wounds. If bruises occur around the entrance of the wound, the ME knows the length of the blade that was used. Bruising indicates a knife plunged to its hilt, so the length of the wound is the length of the knife. Noguchi was once able to exactly describe a murder knife by the wound that it left. He melted a kind of metal and poured it directly into the wound of a young victim of a gang slaying. When the liquid cooled to a solid, Noguchi removed a perfect mold of the murder weapon. He was able to tell the homicide detectives, "It's a knife five and a half inches long, one inch wide, and one sixteenth of an inch thick."[21]

Shooting

Bullet wounds and their patterns provide the medical examiner with even more information than do knife wounds. The ME can identify entrance and exit wounds and tell how closely the weapon was held to the victim's flesh. Entrance wounds are usually circular, with a dark abrasion rim where the bullet scraped the skin. Exit wounds are uneven and have ragged edges. Gunpowder residue—soot and grease from the gunpowder explosion—indicates the distance from which a weapon was fired. When a gun is held hard against the skin, gas and residue are blown into the wound. This is a "tight-contact" wound. A "near-contact" wound is from 1 inch (2.54cm) away and shows residue from the gunpowder, called "fouling," around the wound. A "close-range" wound is from 6 to 10 inches (15 to 25cm) away. Fouling can still be seen on the skin at this range, and stippling is visible, too. Stippling, or tattooing, is caused by powder grains that

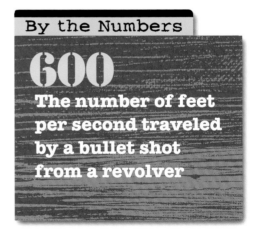

By the Numbers

600

The number of feet per second traveled by a bullet shot from a revolver

are burned and dotted into the skin. An "intermediate-range" wound is from 10 to 36 inches (25 to 91cm) away and shows stippling but no fouling. A "distance-range" wound is 3 feet

(0.91m) or more away, and the wound is clean. Zugibe says, "These wounds produce no tattooing, no soot rings, and no smoke burns, and there is no grease circling the wound."[22] Shapes of bullet wounds vary depending on the distance from which the gun is fired and on whether there is bone underneath the entry point. Tight contact wounds of the scalp, for example, are star shaped. Distance wounds are more likely to be round and small.

Proving Death Was Murder

Knowledge of muzzle-to-target distance helps the medical examiner to determine manner of death. Dix reported a case of a man's body with three gunshot wounds. The murder suspect insisted that the shots were in self-defense, as the victim struggled with him over a gun. The autopsy did not support the suspect's story. One bullet was shot at very close range and had hit the victim's spine. It would have paralyzed him and made him fall. Said Dix, "Thus, it could not have been the first shot as stated by the defendant." The second hole, in the victim's shoulder, showed stippling but no fouling, suggesting it was fired from an intermediate range. The third shot, through the victim's heart, showed stippling and fouling. These patterns suggested the suspect was lying since both close-range wounds were incapacitating and therefore negated the need for more shots. Neither did the exit wound for the third shot support the suspect's statement. The exit wound was a "shored"[23] wound. Instead of being ragged, it was shored up and held together by something solid that supported the skin as the bullet exited. An upright, freely moving victim could not have a shored wound. This proved the victim was lying on the floor when the third shot was fired and killed him. The suspect had not been fighting with the victim when the death occurred. The first shot was really the shoulder wound, incurred as the victim came at the suspect; but the second was to the spine and felled the victim; the third was to the heart while the victim was helpless. Therefore, the death was murder.

Gunshot Wound Patterns

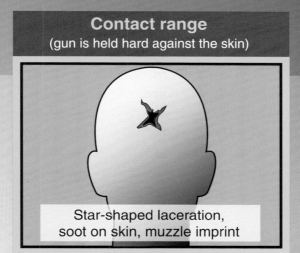

Contact range
(gun is held hard against the skin)

Star-shaped laceration, soot on skin, muzzle imprint

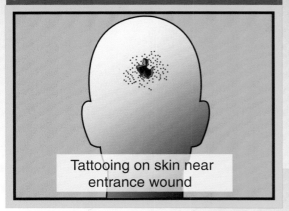

Intermediate range
(gun is held 10 inches to 3 feet from the victim)

Tattooing on skin near entrance wound

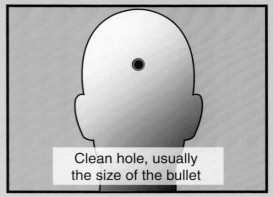

Distance range
(gun is held 3 feet or more from the victim)

Clean hole, usually the size of the bullet

Shining Lights on the Subject

After the medical examiner examines the body for wounds, he or she orders X-rays of the body. X-rays reveal bullets remaining in the victim, bullet fragments, and tips of knives broken off in a body. Next, the ME shines ultraviolet lights on the body in a darkened room. Bodily fluids, such as semen or saliva, glow in ultraviolet light. Bruises not visible to the eye also show up.

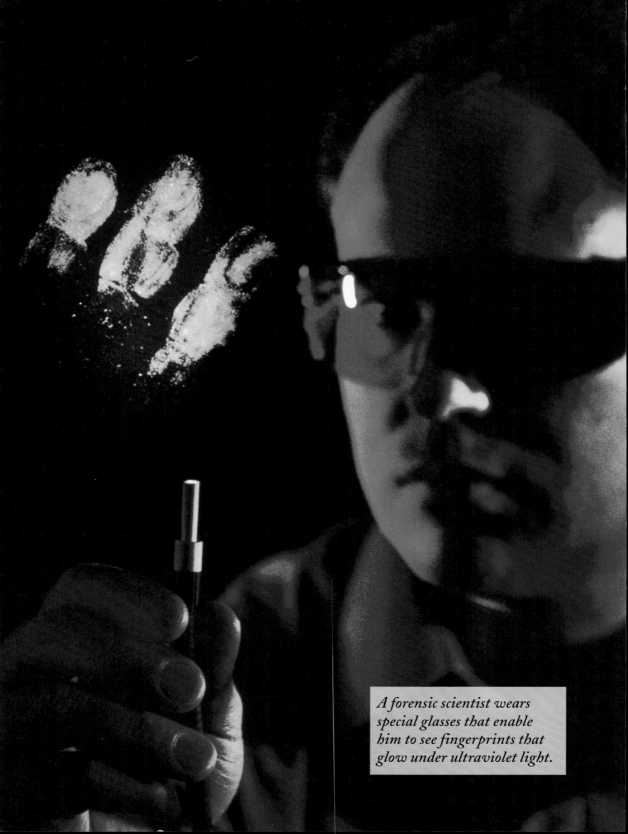

A forensic scientist wears special glasses that enable him to see fingerprints that glow under ultraviolet light.

Zugibe once solved a murder with ultraviolet examination. Liaquat Ali was beaten to death in a robbery. During the autopsy, a large bruise appeared under ultraviolet light. It was the outline of the sole of a shoe. Zugibe measured the outline and figured out the shoe size. With a magnifying glass he discovered the impression of letters in the bruise. They were N, I, and K. Zugibe said,

It's all here before me. Despite the missing last letter, the math is easy to do. . . . Adding an imaginary E to this series, I derive the magic name NIKE, one of the most popular and high-profile brands of sneakers in the world. I inform the police detectives working on the case of this evidence and ask them to bring to the lab any sneakers they can find that are owned by the suspects.[24]

The detectives were able to bring Zugibe a pair of shoes that perfectly matched the bruise and imprint on the victim's body. Zugibe's discovery led to the arrest and conviction of the murderer.

A medical examiner points to metal fragments visible in an X-ray of a victim's skull.

Internal Examination

Even after all the detailed work that a medical examiner does with X-rays, ultraviolet lights, and a magnifying glass, his or her job is far from over. Once the external examination is complete, the medical examiner dissects the corpse and performs the internal examination. Dissection begins with a Y-shaped incision. The first cut goes roughly from shoulder to shoulder.

Then the tail of the Y is cut straight down the body's torso, slightly to one side of the navel. Since the heart is not pumping, just a little blood oozes out. Then the ME cuts the ribs and lays the body open to examination.

All the internal organs are removed and examined for trauma and disease. Any bullets or bullet fragments are recovered and saved for later laboratory evaluation. A blood sample is drawn from the heart and peripheral veins; urine samples are taken; vaginal, oral, and rectal samples are collected in cases where rape is suspected; and thin slices of organ tissue are saved for microscopic examination. The neck is dissected. The ME looks for a fractured larynx or damaged thyroid cartilage and examines the small hyoid bone, which is just above the Adam's apple. Joan D'Alessandro's neck, for instance, showed a hyoid fracture that proved she had been choked to death.

The Last Meal

An organ that gets particular attention in all autopsies is the stomach. Stomach contents can provide important clues about time of death, as well as other information. Baden explains, "Very little interferes with the law of the digestive process. It is not precise to the minute (no biological process is), but within a narrow range of time it is very reliable. Within two hours of eating, 95 percent of the food has moved out of the stomach and into the small intestine. The process stops at death."[25]

Baden's examination of stomach contents was once critical to the conviction of a suspect. David Hendricks's wife and three children were found murdered in their home in November 1983. Hendricks explained to the police that he had taken the children out for pizza around 7:00 P.M. and then seen them to bed around 9:30. He said good-bye to his wife around 10:30 and then left home to catch a midnight plane for a business trip. Someone must have murdered his family during his absence.

When Baden performed the autopsies on the children, he discovered that Hendricks's story did not fit the facts. The stomach contents showed fresh onions and mushrooms, which should have been digested and gone by 9:30 P.M. if the children were still alive. Based on Hendricks's own story, the children were dead when he left on his trip, killed shortly after they returned from their pizza dinner. Said Baden, "The fact that the digestion of all three of the children was the same confirmed their time of death beyond a 95 percent certainty."[26] Hendricks was tried and found guilty of murdering his family.

In another case, in 1986, a Los Angeles medical examiner investigated the stomach contents of a woman who had been strangled. The ME discovered an unusual mixture of foods: mushrooms, water chestnuts, pickles, pepper seeds, and pineapples. She told police detectives about the combination, and they investigated different bars until they found one that served a special drink with these ingredients. Then they found witnesses who told police who had been there with the woman that evening. The murderer was caught.

Telltale Sign of Violence

Hyoid bone

A fractured hyoid bone can indicate that a victim was choked to death.

Into the Skull

When examination of the body organs is finished, the brain is dissected, especially if head wounds are suspected. Baden explains how this is done:

> Once there, I press the blade into the scalp and circumnavigate the skull. This is the second incision to the body. The Y-shaped incision—despite the fact that it is not one continuous cut—is considered the first. The

Autopsy Procedure

1 The ME first examines the outside of the body, looking for obvious clues to the cause of death, such as bullet wounds and strangulation marks. X-rays may be taken.

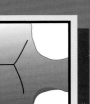

Internal Exam

3 The ME begins the internal exam by making a deep Y incision down the front of the body.

2 The ME also looks for clues that are not so obvious —for example, an odor of almonds around the body could indicate cyanide poisoning, and broken fingernails could mean the victim struggled.

4 The skin, muscle, and soft tissue are peeled back to reveal the abdominal organs and rib cage. The rib cage is cut and lifted out of the body to reveal the heart and lungs.

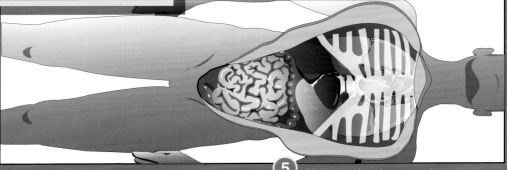

5 After severing the organs' attachment to the spinal cord, the ME removes them.

6 To examine the brain, the ME cuts the skin across the back of the head and pulls the scalp over the face. Then the ME saws off the top of the skull and removes the brain.

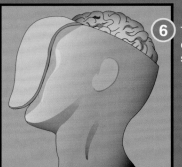

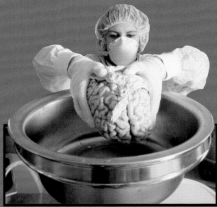

7 Each organ is weighed and examined. Tissue samples and fluids—such as blood, semen, and stomach contents—are sent to the lab for analysis.

scalp incision, ear-to-ear behind the head, is the second. After it is cut, the scalp is then folded so that it will sit like a tight cap over the dead man's closed eyes.[27]

After the cut is finished, the cap of the skull is cut through with a saw and lifted off the head. Then the medical examiner can lift out the brain and examine it. He or she notes where injuries to the brain occur and whether they match injuries to the outside of the head.

It is easy for medical examiners to tell whether a head injury is from a fall or a blow. If an unmoving head is hit by a moving object, such as a hammer, injury to the brain is directly

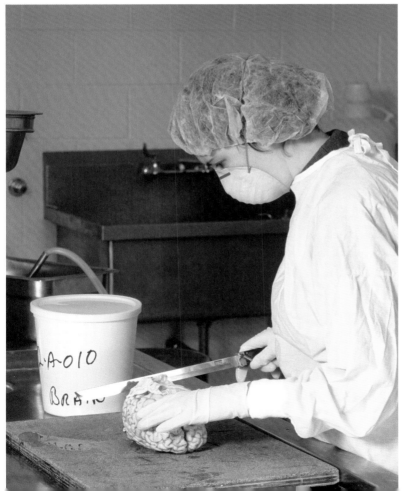

A medical examiner prepares to make cross-sections of a brain.

41

A Moldy Body

Mold may begin to grow on a body in a damp environment. Amazingly, instead of speeding decomposition, mold can actually slow it. Mold naturally absorbs moisture and protects the skin beneath it from the wetness that enables rapid decomposition. Because of this, Florida medical examiner Milton Helpern was able to establish homicide as the manner of death when he performed an autopsy in a 1965 murder case.

Four months after Carmela Coppolino was buried her body was exhumed, and Halpern autopsied the body to look for evidence that she had been poisoned. Water had seeped into the coffin, and the body was covered with mold. When he scraped off the mold, Helpern was able to see a clear needle mark on the skin of a buttock. It was the sign of a drug injection, yet Coppolino had had no medical problems that required shots. Because of this clue, Helpern dissected the brain and sliced off tissue samples for toxicological analysis. Helpern's toxicologist, Joseph Umberger, found evidence of a lethal amount of a drug called succinylcholine in the brain tissue. Court testimony by Helpern and Umberger helped to convict Coppolino's husband, a doctor, of murder.

underneath the bruise or wound on the head. This is called a "coup" injury. If the head was moving, in a fall down the stairs perhaps, the bump on the head does not match the brain injury. The brain is injured on the opposite side from the head wound. This happens because the brain floats a little in the skull and is driven against the opposite side in a natural fall, as when the back of the head strikes the pavement in an accident. This kind of injury is called "contra-coup."

One medical examiner proved that a presumed fall from a bridge was actually a homicide by discovering a coup injury. Police had found a homeless man lying under a bridge and assumed he had either fallen or committed suicide by jumping off the bridge. The medical examiner did an autopsy of the man's brain. He found bruised and damaged brain tissue directly beneath the skull fracture on the man's head. There was no contra-coup injury. Dix explains, "Thus the pathologist reasoned that the man was in a stationary position relative to the moving object which struck him. That is, someone hit him in the head."[28]

Closing Up

After examining the brain and taking tissue samples, the medical examiner is ready to close the body up again. Organs are returned, usually in a bag placed in the abdominal cavity, and the head and body incisions are sewn up. Then the body can be released to the family for burial. The medical examiner writes a detailed report of the findings but is not yet ready to consider the autopsy complete. Laboratory tests and examinations of all the collected blood, tissue samples, and trace evidence must be done. Only when the medical examiner has the results of these investigations will a final autopsy report be issued and signed.

Poison, Blood, and DNA

In forensic laboratories around the country, specialized scientists work under the direction of a chief medical examiner and use their knowledge and skill to examine autopsy evidence and help investigate cause of death. David Fisher, a forensic scientist with the New York City medical examiner's office, says, "You can't help but have a deep sense of satisfaction when your work helps put some bad guy behind bars or helps release someone who's innocent and has already been wrongly imprisoned."[29] Forensic scientists may examine bloodstains from clothing or scrapings from under fingernails. Some analyze the blood, bodily fluids, and tissue samples collected during an autopsy. Still others, such as Fisher, use DNA fingerprinting to match a suspect to evidence on the victim.

Microscopic Investigation

Much autopsy evidence is examined with microscopes. Microscopes can reveal petechiae in body tissues, for example. These small hemorrhages appear in lungs as well as eyes when a victim is smothered or strangled. When Gilbert microscopically examined the lungs of one of the children who died in the Pankow case, she found many petechial hemorrhages.

In cases of suspected drowning, microscopes are used to search bone samples for minute single-celled creatures called diatoms that live in water. A medical examiner may be suspicious, for example, that a body found in a lake was killed elsewhere and dumped in the water. If the victim drowned, diatoms should be present in the body. D.P. Lyle, a medical doctor and forensic author, says, "If the victim's heart is still beating when she inhales the water, any diatoms in the water pass

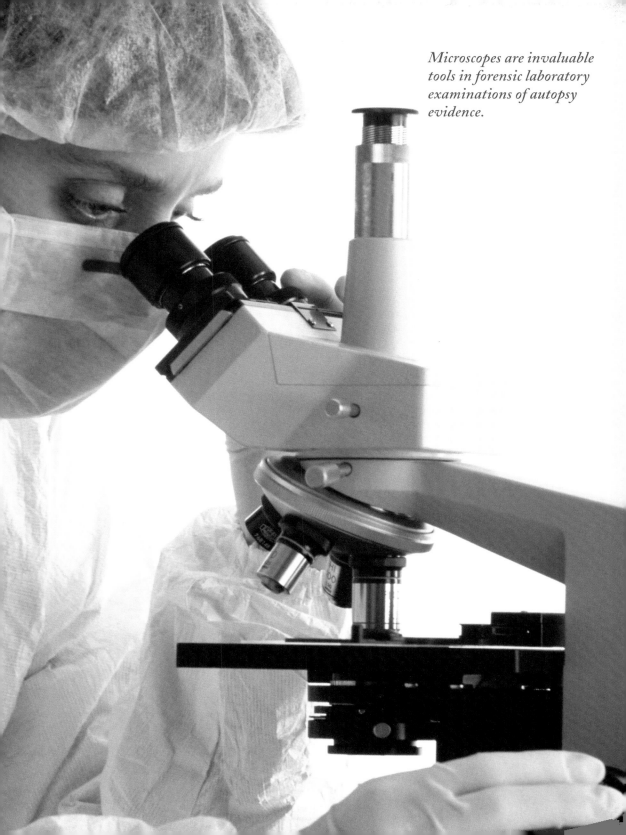

Microscopes are invaluable tools in forensic laboratory examinations of autopsy evidence.

through the lungs, enter the blood stream, and are pumped throughout the body. They tend to collect in the bone marrow. Microscopic analysis may reveal diatoms, meaning the victim was alive when she entered the water, instead of being placed there after death."[30] The absence of diatoms may suggest that a homicide was committed.

When regular light microscopes are not powerful enough to investigate bodily evidence, scientists use scanning electron microscopes (SEMs). Lyle explains how they work: "A standard microscope uses light for viewing an object, but an SEM uses an electron beam. This beam sweeps across the object and is viewed through electromagnetic lenses that greatly magnify the image and provide incredible clarity."[31] SEMs magnify images up to one hundred thousand times. They can see a single virus or search the individual parts of a blood cell for

A scanning electron microscope can produce images of tiny structures, such as the cells lining a blood vessel in lung tissue (inset).

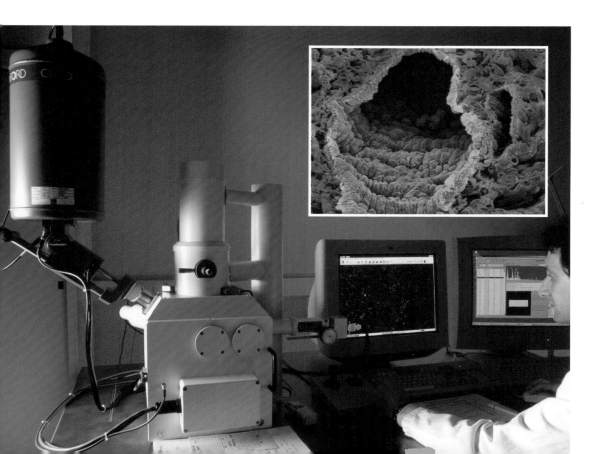

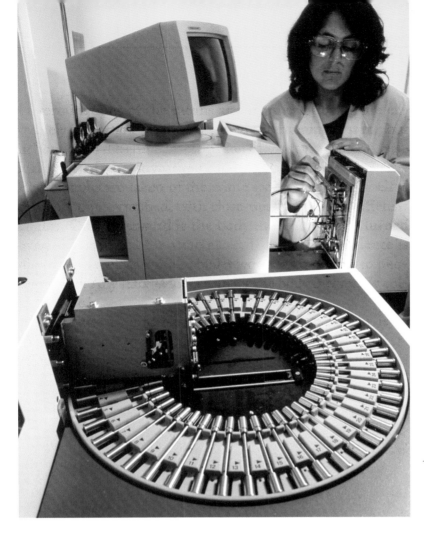

A gas chromatograph checks blood and tissue samples for toxins.

injury. They make it possible to analyze gunpowder particles on skin and match them to a particular ammunition.

GC/MS Examination

Another useful investigative tool in the forensics laboratory is the gas chromatograph (GC) with mass spectrometer (MS). Crime writer Katherine Ramsland calls this combination "the real workhorse of a crime lab."[32] With GC/MS analysis, blood and other body tissues can be tested for the presence of poison, drugs, or any other foreign chemical that could cause death or impairment. The medical examiner simply has to know what chemical to ask the lab to search for. A blood or other sample

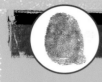

Searching for Harmful Chemicals

A GC/MS analysis identifies substances that may have caused harm or death. The process works this way:

1 **A chemical mixture,** such as a blood sample, is injected into one end of a column or glass tube where it is heated and turned into a gas.

2 **Inside the column** is a carrier gas, usually helium, into which the sample gas is swept. Each compound in the sample speeds through the coiled tube at a different rate because each has a different weight.

3 **The various substances** are separated by their rate of travel.

4 **Each substance** then moves through a second chamber where it is bombarded with electrons that break up the substance into fragments and molecules.

5 **The fragments** are passed through an electric or magnetic field that filters and separates them according to their masses.

6 **Then the elements** enter a detector that sends data about the mass of each substance to a computer and translates it into readable results on a graph.

7 **Each element** has a different mass and a different pattern of fragments, and the computer holds a library of thousands of these substance patterns. Scientists can identify every substance by comparing its mass to the known mass and fragment pattern of any element or compound stored in the computer.

from the autopsy is heated until it becomes a gas. This gas is bombarded with electrons so that it is broken into individual molecules. Then the molecules are sped through a coiled glass tube. Every element travels at a different speed, and the molecules of each element have a different weight. A computerized detector identifies each element present in the blood by its speed of travel. The weight and energy of each element are automatically analyzed to figure the amount of each element in the blood sample.

The GC/MS gives scientists an automatic readout of the poisons or foreign elements in a blood sample. Scientists can tell how much methamphetamine, for instance, is in the blood. They can also find poisons, or even tell if a natural chemical in the body, such as insulin, occurs in a normal amount. Insulin, like almost any substance, is healthy and valuable in a small amount but lethal, or toxic, if the quantity is too large. Huge amounts of water can be toxic; too much pure oxygen can be fatal. All medicines can be toxic in large amounts. As Lyle explains, "The right dose is medication; the wrong dose is poison."[33] Toxicologic investigation provides the medical examiner with precise, accurate information about the levels of many substances in the blood or tissue of a body.

Toxicology Says Murder

In one suspicious death Noguchi used toxicology analysis to demonstrate not only that a homicide had occurred, but how it occurred. A man was injured in a car accident and was recovering in the hospital. His uncle, who had been driving the car, sat beside him, seemingly quite concerned for his nephew's welfare. No one knew that the uncle held a large life insurance policy on his nephew's life. After the uncle left for the day, his nephew suddenly went into a coma. Despite the best efforts of his doctors, the nephew died. His injuries had not been that severe, but doctors had only suspicions and no evidence of a homicide.

Noguchi did the autopsy, expecting to find evidence of poison, but there were no needle marks on the nephew's body and no poisons in his blood. Noguchi visited the hospital and examined the crime scene. Suddenly he realized that the IV the doctors had used to treat the nephew could be the way that a poison was introduced. Microscopic inspection revealed a needle mark on the IV tubing. Noguchi said, "So now we knew how the uncle had injected the nephew. But since no poison or drug had been in the nephew's body, we still did not know what had killed him."[34] The answer had to be a toxic amount of a naturally occurring substance. Then police discovered that the uncle had worked in a hospital where he administered insulin to patients. Noguchi ordered toxicology tests, which revealed a huge, fatal amount of insulin in the nephew's blood samples. The uncle was convicted of murder.

In one case, a woman used fentanyl, a drug medical examiners rarely test for, to kill her husband.

An Almost Perfect Crime

GC/MS analysis identifies the smallest traces of chemicals in body samples, but only if the medical examiner or toxicologists search for those chemicals. Kristin Rossum, an assistant toxicologist in the San Diego County Medical Examiner's Office, knew this. She tried to get away with murder by using a rare and unusual poison, stolen from the toxicology lab. It was a chemical for which medical examiners ordinarily do not search when they autopsy a suspected poisoning victim. The medical examiner and another toxicology lab in Los Angeles, however, were not fooled.

NDC 50458-036-05   One (100µg/h) System   CII
DURAGESIC 100µg/h
(FENTANYL TRANSDERMAL SYSTEM)
In vivo delivery of 100µg/h fentanyl for 72 hours
NOT FOR ACUTE OR POSTOPERATIVE USE
Each transdermal system contains:
10mg fentanyl and 0.4ml alcohol USP
KEEP OUT OF REACH OF CHILDREN
Rx only
00085002   5000510
JANSSEN   PHARMACEUTICA PRODUCTS, L.P.
ATTENTION: Only for use by patient for whom prescribed.

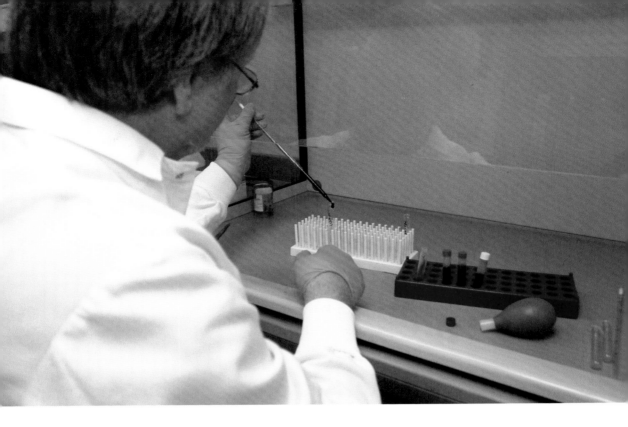

Rossum was married to Gregory de Villers. When de Villers was found dead in 2000 police assumed it was suicide by drug overdose. He lay on the floor of his bedroom, covered with rose petals, with his wife's journal beside him. In the journal Rossum had written that she wanted to leave her husband for another man—her boss in the toxicology laboratory, Michael Robertson. Rossum told police that de Villers became severely depressed when he found out she was leaving him. De Villers's brother, however, refused to believe that the death was a suicide. He insisted that the police investigate the possibility of murder.

An investigation at the San Diego County Medical Examiner's Office revealed missing drugs. One of these drugs, called fentanyl, is rarely used. It is so powerful that it is given only to dying cancer patients. The drug was stored in a drug locker to which Robertson had the key. Brian Blackbourne, the medical examiner in San Diego, sent tissue samples from de Villers's autopsy to a toxicology lab in Los Angeles. He did

A toxicologist prepares a blood sample to test it for poison.

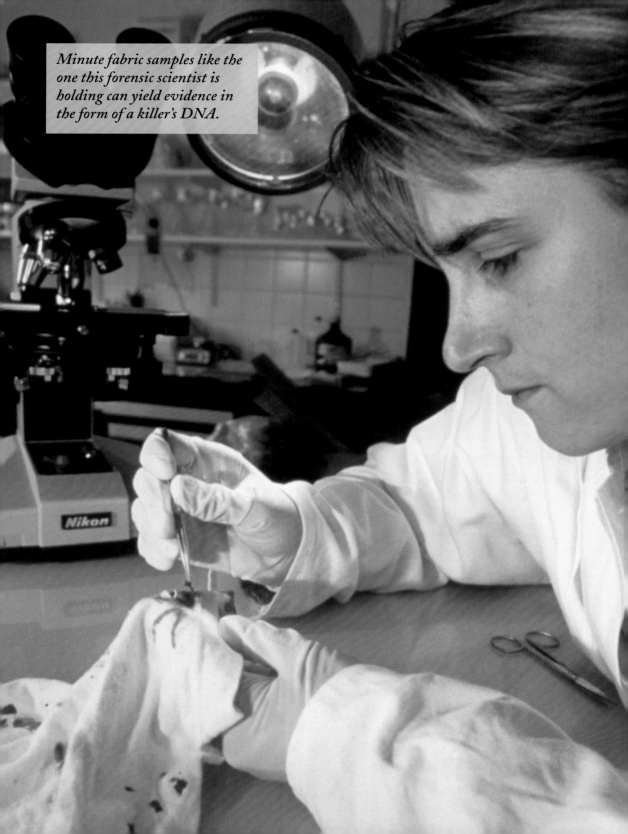

Minute fabric samples like the one this forensic scientist is holding can yield evidence in the form of a killer's DNA.

not want his own toxicology lab to be trusted with the tests, but he wanted the samples to be tested for fentanyl. In de Villers's tissue, Los Angeles toxicologists found seven times the amount of fentanyl that it would take to kill someone.

The medical examiner's office fired Rossum and Robertson. Robertson went back to his native Australia. Rossum was arrested for murdering her husband with fentanyl sneaked from the toxicology lab. At the trial the prosecutor told the jury that Rossum had arranged the crime scene to look like a suicide. She had even sprinkled the rose petals on her husband as he lay unconscious. "It was the perfect poison,"[35] said assistant district attorney David Hendron. However, the drug was not quite perfect. Once toxicologists knew what to look for, the fentanyl was identified. Rossum maintained her innocence, but the toxicology evidence was too strong for the jury. Rossum was convicted of murder in 2002.

The DNA Story

Toxicology is not the only function of forensics laboratories. DNA experts are skilled at identifying suspects by using blood and biological evidence collected during the autopsy. Any suspicious blood or fluid evidence collected by the medical examiner is sent to the lab to be tested for a DNA match. The trace evidence may point to the murderer. When Zugibe matched the Nike sneakers to the bruise on the beating victim's body, he also discovered traces of blood embedded in the shoes. He sent a swab of this blood along with a sample of the victim's blood to the DNA lab. The victim's blood matched the blood on the shoes, proving that the owner of the sneakers had been at the crime scene. When performed correctly, DNA fingerprinting is a scientific method of matching

DNA (shown in this computer-generated model) can be used to tie a killer to a victim or to a crime scene.

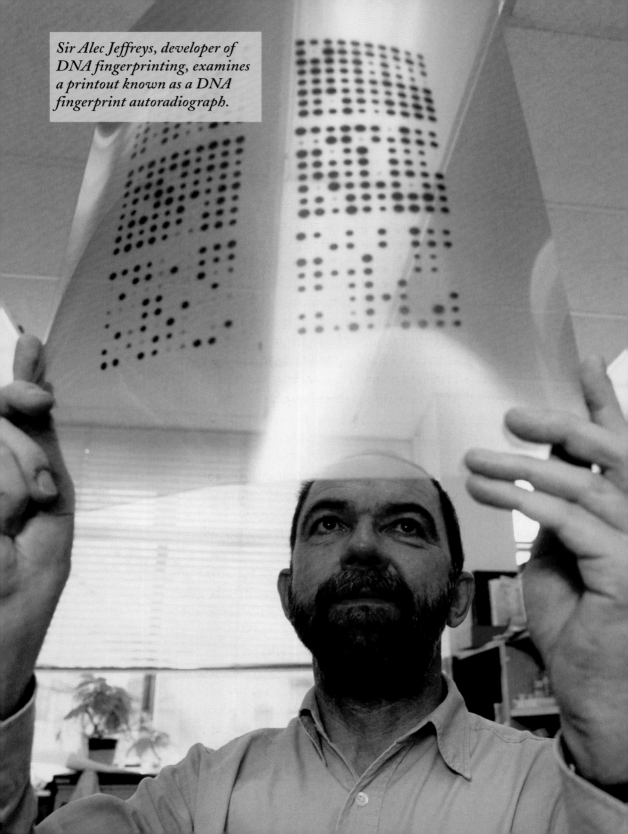

Sir Alec Jeffreys, developer of DNA fingerprinting, examines a printout known as a DNA fingerprint autoradiograph.

one tissue or fluid sample to another with unquestionable accuracy.

DNA stands for deoxyribonucleic acid. It is the genetic information within the cells that determines how every living thing develops and functions. Human bodies are made of trillions of cells. In the nucleus of each cell are the chromosomes, made up of long strings of DNA. The DNA spells out a code, like the letters of a giant book of instructions. DNA is arranged as a long, twisted, spiraling ladder. The rungs, or bases, of the ladder are the letters that form chemical messages.

The four letters in the DNA alphabet are A (the chemical called adenine), T (thymine), G (guanine), and C (cytosine). At each rung of the ladder, A can join only with T to make a rung, and G hooks with C. Every human has about 3 billion such base pairs in his or her DNA, but they can be strung together in differing orders up the ladder. A long string, or sequence, of the rungs of the ladder forms a gene, and that gene spells out chemical directions to the body. Because of DNA, people come in many different shapes and sizes, have different hair and eye color, and even develop different diseases.

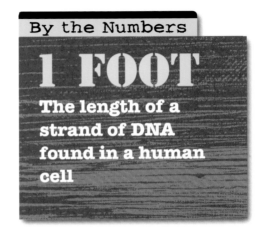

By the Numbers

1 FOOT

The length of a strand of DNA found in a human cell

Junk DNA: Different for Everyone

Although most DNA in an individual body is identical to that of other humans, the way some strings are arranged is unique to each person. Outside the genes are many strands of DNA that have no known function. Scientists call this DNA "junk DNA." Junk DNA base pairs can repeat themselves over and over, at many different DNA sites, in different sequences in different people. The unique pattern of these repeating sequences, called polymorphisms, is each person's DNA fingerprint. For example, the base pair AT may be repeated in one person as ATAT, while another may have the repeated sequence of ATATATAT. AT is repeated twice for the first person and four times for the second. A third person may have five repeats, but a fourth may have sixteen. These sequences are called "tandem repeats." Although many people may share some identical tandem repeats, no one except identical twins has the same pattern of repeats at all the sites on the DNA ladder that DNA experts can examine. Like fingerprints, the polymorphisms are unique to each individual. DNA experts say that the chance of one person's DNA profile matching another's approaches less than one in trillions.

DNA Profiling

In the DNA laboratory, scientists test for DNA matches between two different tissue or blood samples. If the blood on a shoe matches the blood of a victim, for example, there is really no chance that the blood came from someone else. DNA testing to identify the unique pattern of tandem repeats in a sample and create a profile is a complicated technique that involves careful laboratory analysis, mathematical formulas, and computer technology. The most common procedure is known as PCR/STR (polymerase chain reaction/short tandem repeats).

With this technique, a sample is first broken down with a chemical that releases the DNA from the cells. The next step is often the PCR procedure, which is a way to replicate and multiply the DNA in a sample until it is large enough to be tested conveniently and efficiently in the laboratory. Scientists then use an enzyme, a special chemical, to cut up the DNA into fragments at known short tandem repeat sites. The sites that are not repeat sites are digested by the enzyme. The resulting fragments represent short repeats, for example ATAT, at different sites on the DNA ladder. The fragments are placed in a special gel and subjected to an electric current. This current sorts the fragments by size, from shortest to longest. Special chemically fluorescent tags are attached to the fragments so they can be seen. The length of each fragment can then be measured, and the fragments are lined up in a readout that

An Alternative DNA Test

Television crime shows often leave the impression that any biological trace evidence left behind by a criminal contains DNA. This is not quite true. Almost all body cells contain DNA, but red blood cells and hairs have no nuclei and so do not have nuclear DNA—the only kind that yields a DNA fingerprint. In the case of a blood sample, the lack of nuclear DNA does not matter because white blood cells do have nuclear DNA. Once a blood sample is appropriately collected, it can be used to develop a DNA profile and identify a murderer with unquestionable accuracy.

Hairs, however, can present a problem. They have nuclei and nuclear DNA only in their roots. If a rootless hair is discovered at a crime scene, no DNA fingerprinting is possible. Investigators must use another, less-accurate DNA profiling technique in the search for a suspect. This technique uses mtDNA (mitochondrial DNA), which is outside the nucleus of the cell. MtDNA is attached to each cell's mitochondria—the cell's power generators. Because humans inherit mtDNA, unchanged, from their mothers, it can be used to create a profile that can then be matched to family members. MtDNA cannot distinguish between brothers and sisters and does not yield a true DNA profile. It can point to a suspect, but cannot identify any one at certainties of billions to one as is possible with nuclear DNA.

looks like a bar code on a package in the grocery store. This picture is a series of DNA bands of different sizes that can be compared to the bands in a second sample. If the bands are the same, the lab has a match.

Medical examiners and forensic investigators can get DNA samples for STR testing from all sorts of trace evidence. At the scene of the crime, investigators may collect a discarded cigarette butt or a used drinking cup. During the autopsy the ME may collect semen from a victim's vagina, hairs or blood drops on the victim's clothing, or skin from under fingernails. All these sources contain cells with DNA that tell the story of the crime to the forensic laboratories. Zugibe says, "We can run from the forensic pathologist. We can hide from the forensic pathologist. But we can never entirely disappear."[36]

DNA Never Lies

Members of law enforcement agencies use kits like this one to collect and identify blood samples, which are analyzed for their DNA content.

Murderers may deny their involvement in a crime, but DNA evidence often finds them out. When Alan and Diane Johnson were shot to death in their bedroom in 2003, DNA evidence implicated their sixteen-year-old daughter, Sarah. Sarah's parents disapproved of her new boyfriend, and police believed that she killed them so she could be with him. Sarah insisted that she was innocent. She claimed an intruder must have entered her parents' bedroom and killed them. However, DNA evi-

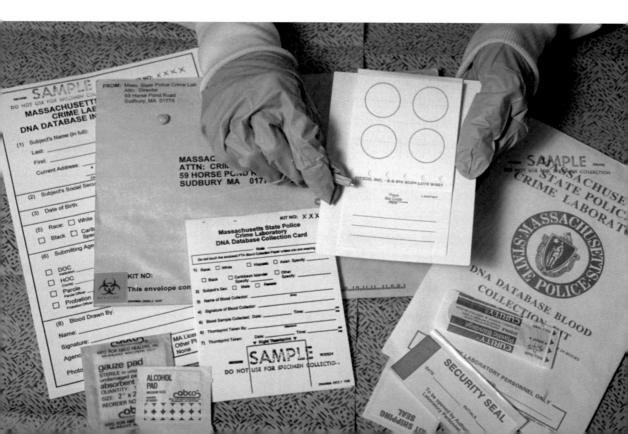

dence linked Sarah to the crime. Blood found on Sarah's pink bathrobe matched the Johnsons' blood. Blood on Sarah's socks matched Diane Johnson's blood. A glove thrown into the garbage carried DNA from Sarah. Two bullet cartridges found in Sarah's bedroom held Diane Johnson's DNA. Sarah claimed she had not gone into her parents' bedroom, but the DNA evidence said otherwise. Along with the gun residue found on Sarah's bathrobe, the trace evidence was enough for a jury. Sarah was convicted of killing her parents in 2005. Even Sarah's family believed she was guilty. Her aunt asked, "How can you deny doing this in the face of such overwhelming evidence?"[37]

The DNA Bank

DNA typing and sample matches have solved many homicides, even years-old ones called "cold cases." Since the introduction of PCR technology, murders have been reinvestigated, and murderers have been caught, thanks to DNA matches. Today, the FBI maintains a national database, the Combined DNA Information System (CODIS). DNA profiles of convicted criminals are stored at CODIS, as is DNA evidence found at crime scenes. Forensic investigators and pathologists around the country can submit DNA profiles to the database and search for a known match. By 2004 CODIS had made more than seventeen thousand matches, or "hits," and helped investigate more than twenty thousand crimes.

DNA and a Cold Case

One of those cases was the murder of Mia Zapata, a rock singer who was raped and strangled in Seattle, Washington, in 1993. Police had no clues to help them solve the murder. As the years went by, her father said, "I came to accept the fact that it was never going to be solved."[38] In 2002, however, police investigators working on cold cases made an important discovery. The medical examiner who did the autopsy on Zapata had collected and frozen a small sample of saliva found on her body. At that time the medical examiner was unable to test the saliva for DNA. PCR techniques were not yet invented, and the sample was too small for the DNA testing procedures then available. With the hope that someday the sample would be useful, the ME saved the sample in his lab.

In 2002 police sent the saliva sample to Jodi Sass, a DNA expert at the Washington State crime lab. With modern technology, she was able to develop a DNA profile, which she submitted to CODIS. CODIS found a match. The DNA from Zapata's body belonged to Jesus Mezquia, who lived in Florida. Mezquia denied ever having met Zapata, but the police investigators trusted their evidence. Said one, "There's no way that saliva could be where it was and him not have any knowledge of who this lady was."[39]

Mezquia was arrested and brought to Washington for trial. When Zapata's father heard the news, he exclaimed, "I couldn't believe it. I couldn't believe it. . . . It's a miracle. But we think we've got him."[40] In 2004 Mezquia was found guilty of killing Mia Zapata. DNA profiling had solved another cold case.

The forensic scientists who analyze the DNA and blood evidence collected by medical examiners are invaluable members of homicide investigative teams. Without them, many murders would go unsolved.

CHAPTER 4

Decomposition

Bodies without heads, rotting bodies, mummified bodies—such situations challenge the medical examiner in unique ways. Cause and manner of death may be obscured. Even the identity of the body may be in doubt. Still, although their investigations are not always successful, MEs can accomplish remarkable things with these corpses.

A Mangled Corpse

Even with a mutilated body a careful autopsy can reveal the cause and manner of death. Luv Sharma and his colleagues were medical examiners at a forensics department in India. They described an autopsy in which they proved that a presumed suicide was really murder. The body of a young man was found on the railroad tracks after it was run over by a train. Police took the body to a local hospital, where a doctor examined it and said the death was either an accident or suicide. The man's father did not believe it and requested a complete autopsy. The body was sent to Sharma's facility.

Sharma noted, "The body was received in 7 separate parts." On the autopsy table lay a torso with part of a head. A large part of the skull was torn off and rested nearby. The severed arms and legs lay there, too, as well as one hand separated from its arm. Sharma paid particular attention to the edges of the severed body parts. He noticed that no blood had been absorbed by the fibers of the bones. This proved to him that the body had been cut by the train wheels after the man was already dead. Otherwise, the heart's pumping would have sent blood into the bones. The case was not a suicide. Then Sharma examined the torso as best he could. He found bruises around

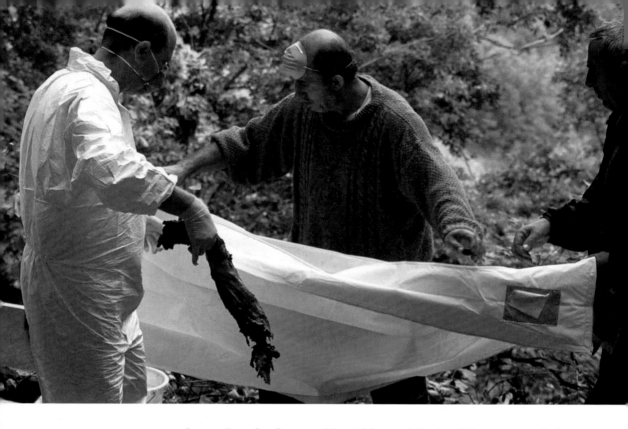

Forensic experts place the decomposed remains of a homicide victim in a body bag.

the neck and a fractured hyoid bone. Much of the chest and abdomen showed large bruises, too. When Sharma checked the stomach contents, he found a brown fluid that the toxicology lab identified as poison. Sharma said, "Thus with the detailed examination of the body, it was concluded that the deceased had first been poisoned, then throttled, and his dead body was laid in a railway track to get transected by a train."[41] Sharma's determination of homicide led to a police investigation that found the group of men who had committed the murder.

Rotting Corpses

Sharma's autopsy yielded a lot of information, even though the body was in pieces. Sometimes, however, a body lies undiscovered for a long time. Then an autopsy is even more difficult than with a mangled body, because the corpse has decomposed. Zugibe explains, "'Decomposition,' in brief, is a blandly neutral word for a universally abhorrent and unpalatable reality: rotting; or, to be even more graphic, being eaten." After death the bacteria that naturally occur in a person's body begin to eat the corpse's tissues. The digestive juices in the stomach, with no food to digest, digest the body instead. Bacteria from outside the body enter the corpse and attack the tissues as well. These microscopic organisms eat at the flesh, eventually reducing it from a solid to a liquid. This process is known as putrefaction. Zugibe adds, "Even a few hours after death, the inside of a corpse becomes a teeming sea of scavengers."[42]

Decomposition begins about four minutes after death, starting in the inside and working outward in five distinct stages. At temperatures below about 70°F (21°C) little decay is visible in the first two or three days. This first stage is called "fresh." It starts at the moment of death and ends when the second stage, or bloat, begins. The first sign of bloat is a greenish discoloration on the skin of the abdomen that spreads to the chest and thighs and eventually down the limbs. Within a week the abdomen starts to swell, or bloat, from all the gases produced by the bacteria. The skin color changes from green to purple to black. Within about two or three weeks after death skin begins to blister, and fluids ooze out of the

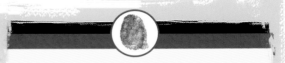

Flames in Vain

Murderers sometimes try to obscure the evidence of their crimes by burning the body. These efforts rarely succeed. Fires outside of crematoria do not burn hot enough to destroy a body or wipe out evidence of homicide. In his 2005 book Dissecting Death *Frederick Zugibe explains what fire really does to a body:*

What actually happens at such relatively low temperatures, however—around 1200°F (648.9°C)—is that instead of disintegrating, the corpse's flesh roasts much in the manner of, if you will forgive the gruesome analogy, meat on a backyard barbecue.

From your own kitchen experience you probably know that if a cut or chop from the butcher counter is left on a flame for many hours, the meat does not turn to ashes. Quite to the contrary, it forms a hard, crusty shell that keeps the core of the meat intact. Ironically, burning flesh over a wood flame does not destroy it. It cooks it, protects it, and most of all, preserves it.

nose and mouth, as the whole body puffs up with gas. At the end of this stage, says forensic scientist M. Lee Goff, "the corpse looks somewhat like a balloon."[43]

The third stage of decomposition is decay. Zugibe explains, "After three or more weeks pass, a body starts to come apart in earnest."[44] Organs such as the brain and intestines liquefy, the outer skin peels off in huge chunks, and hair and fingernails fall out. The gas escapes the body, and the corpse deflates. Gradually, the body breaks open like an overripe tomato, and flesh disintegrates.

By the end of the decay stage only skin, cartilage, and bones remain, along with a few tough body organs such as the heart and uterus. Thus begins the post-decay or "dry" stage. In this stage the skin and remaining tissues decay until only bones and hair are left. Once that happens, the corpse is in the skeletal

Skeletal remains, such as this skull and teeth, can last for years.

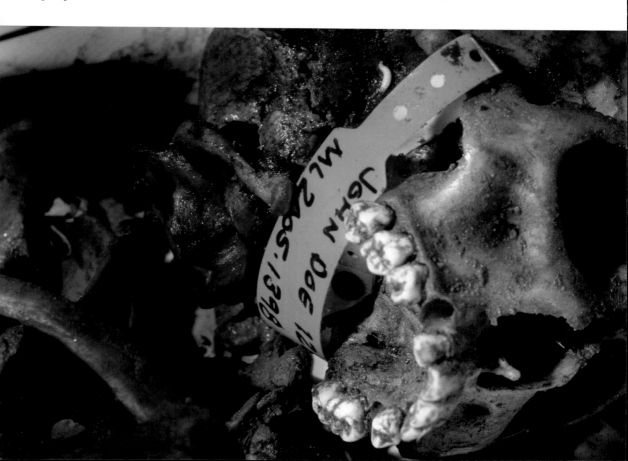

stage. Goff says, "There is no definite end to this stage of decomposition."[45] Depending on the environment and weather conditions, skeletons may last for years.

Hot and Cold, Wet and Dry

Stages of decomposition can yield clues about time of death, but a body's decay is not very predictable. Corpses in hot environments decay more quickly than those in cold places. A body left outdoors will be attacked by many different animals and insects that gnaw and scatter bones and eat up flesh quite quickly. When a body is in water, fish and algae do the same thing, and the fat in the body is slowly turned into a kind of soap that coats the outsides. In a dry coffin, however, decomposition can be slowed and delayed for decades. In a very hot, dry environment, such as a desert, bodies may dry out instead of decomposing and become natural mummies. Mummification stops putrefaction.

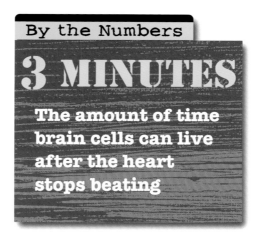

By the Numbers

3 MINUTES

The amount of time brain cells can live after the heart stops beating

Putrefying Clues

The variables of decomposition can make an autopsy difficult. A body that is badly decayed may be barely recognizable as human. Zugibe says,

> In real life, a bloated, blackened body, especially one that has been worked over by insects, forest animals, and vermin, is so altered that it is difficult not only to identify the person, but to tell what color, race, and even sex they once happened to be.

Still, there is the mandate: Use every scientific means available to find out everything possible, especially time of death, even if you know in advance that the value of these tests is limited.[46]

Forensic workers sometimes must rely on the DNA extracted from tissue samples to identify a body.

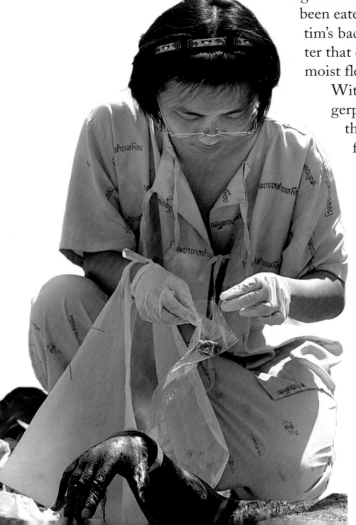

That was the goal of medical examiner Charles Odom when he autopsied a decomposed body in Honolulu in 1984. The woman's body was found lying partly in a water-filled ditch. The head was just a skull; its jaw had come loose and lay a few feet away from the body. One hand was missing; the other hand was dried up and mummified. Internal organs were gone, and most of the chest had been eaten away by insects. Only the victim's back, which had been lying in water that delayed decomposition, still had moist flesh attached.

Without its face or hands with fingerprints, Odom could not identify the corpse. He needed help from forensic dentistry. He ordered X-rays of the teeth in the jaw. Then a forensic dentist compared the corpse's teeth to dental X-rays from a woman previously reported missing. The dental X-rays matched, giving Odom an identification for the victim. He autopsied what was left of the body as best he could and discovered that the hyoid bone in the throat was fractured. Now he knew the manner of death—homicide by strangulation. Still, the story of the death was very incomplete. Odom made a decision that was quite unusual and forward thinking for 1984. He looked at the insect life crawling on the rotting flesh and decided to call in a bug scientist, a forensic entomologist, to help him establish the time of death.

Time to Eat

M. Lee Goff was an expert on flies, maggots, and beetles and had special knowledge about how bugs feed on decomposing bodies. He came to the morgue and collected maggots—the wormlike young of flies—that were still feeding on decaying flesh. He found some beetles eating the skin. He also collected empty pupal cases, which are like the cocoons of butterflies, that were attached to the body's ribs. He took these samples back to his own laboratory so he could try to help the medical examiner tell this body's story. Goff put the maggots in a special rearing chamber and gave them liver to eat. He watched the maggots develop, first growing larger, then forming pupae, and finally emerging as adult flies. He was then able to identify each kind of fly. From his experience, he already knew the behavior and life cycle of the kinds of flies that feed on corpses. He knew when each arrived, how long it took to lay eggs, what part of the body the maggots ate, and how many days it took for each maggot to become an adult fly. Once his maggots had grown to adulthood, he not only knew what kind of flies they were, he also could figure out when each had invaded the body.

The empty pupae and some maggots were from blowflies. Blowflies feed only on moist, soft flesh, and their maggots were only on the part of the body that had been in the water. In Hawaii, blowflies begin to feed on flesh ten minutes after death. They lay eggs on the body for six days, and then the flies depart. When the eggs hatch, the maggots feed and develop into adult flies in eleven days. So these maggots and empty pupae gave Goff a minimal time since death of seventeen days. The time was not completely certain since water can affect decomposition, but it was close.

The First Use of Forensic Entomology

In France, in 1855, a doctor named Bergeret (no one knows his first name) became the first westerner to use forensic entomology to solve a crime. A baby's body had been found stuffed behind the bricks of a boardinghouse chimney. Police did not know whether to arrest the current boarder or someone else. Bergeret noticed some moth larvae crawling on the body. He took these larvae back to his office and grew them to adulthood. He reasoned that he could learn exactly how many days the baby had been dead if he counted the days his adult moths took to lay eggs and added that number to the days it took for the larvae to grow to the size of those on the baby's body. Bergeret was successful, and police were able to find the woman who had lived in the room at the time the baby died. The woman admitted to hiding the baby's body behind the chimney but said the baby had been born dead. She placed it behind the chimney because she could not afford a burial. At her trial, she was found not guilty of murder.

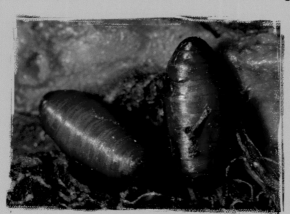

The larvae and pupae of insects that invade a corpse can be clues to when a victim died.

Goff also found cheese skipper maggots on the body, but these maggots do not attack a corpse until several days after death. The size of the cheese skipper maggots told him that the body had been decomposing for nineteen days. The maggots could not have hatched from eggs and grown to their current size any sooner than that.

The beetles were hide beetles that are attracted to a corpse only when it reaches the post-decay stage and is dry. Goff knew that hide beetles do not attack a body in Hawaii until eleven days after decomposition begins. These beetles had laid eggs that had hatched into young, called larvae. The larvae were eight days old. Given the life cycle of hide beetles, the corpse had been decaying for nineteen days.

Goff put all his bug facts together and told Odom that his best estimate of how long the body had been decomposing was nineteen days. Odom included the estimate in his final autopsy report. It was one of the first times that an ME had used the science of forensic entomology in an investigation. With the information about time of death, police investigators were able to identify the man last seen with the victim and bring him to trial for her murder. Goff remarked, "The suspect was convicted of second degree murder and the major witnesses were flies."[47]

A forensic entomologist carefully removes insects from a body in an effort to estimate the time of death.

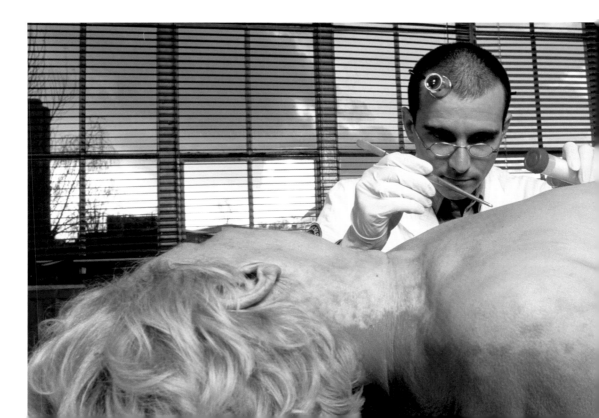

How Insects Invade a Corpse

1 **The pioneer flies** are the first to discover a dead body, within minutes after a death. They are house flies of the family Muscidae and blowflies of the family Calliphoridae. They eat flesh and lay their eggs in body openings.

2 **Next come** the flesh flies called Sarcophagidae. As their name implies, these flies eat soft flesh.

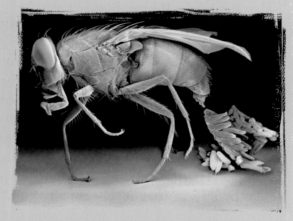

Blowflies, such as this one depositing eggs, are often among the first insects to begin feeding on a corpse.

3 **A blowfly** called *Chrysomya rufifacies* arrives after the other flies and eats their maggots as well as the body flesh.

4 **As the soft flesh** is eaten away and the body begins to dry out, two other flies appear. They are the cheese flies of the family Piophilidae and the coffin flies known scientifically as Phoridae.

5 **Many different** kinds of beetles and mites show up. Along with cheese flies and coffin flies, they finish the job of cleaning up the bones.

Body Identification

Flies may tell a medical examiner the time of death, but they cannot identify a body. Victim identification is an important part of a medical examiner's job. Without an identification, the cause of death and the perpetrator may never be discovered. With decaying bodies even DNA testing may be useless. A DNA profile cannot identify anyone unless there is a known sample to match it against. Dental records are of no value either if the victim's dentist is not already known. As Baden says, "Good as they are, neither DNA nor dental work comes with a return address label."[48] Often, fingerprints are the best method for identifying a body, since fingerprint records of average citizens are commonly available.

Once in a while decomposition can actually help the medical examiner get fingerprints. In the decay stage skin slips off bodies easily. Baden explains, "In some decomposed bodies, the outermost layer of skin on the hand will deglove—literally come off—and you just need to put your own gloved finger into it and roll off a print or two."[49] Usually, though, more effort is needed to get fingerprints from a long-dead corpse.

Mummified Fingers

Zugibe once was brought a woman's body that had been discovered on a remote mountainside. The body was mummified, and the hands were shriveled and hard. The autopsy showed that the woman had been strangled, but Zugibe could not identify her. He remembers, "We tried every means at our disposal to identify the body: dental charting, dental x-rays, full body x-rays, anthropological studies, hair studies, artist drawings, and descriptive profiling. The gathered information was sent to law enforcement and missing persons agencies, but to no avail."[50]

Usually, medical examiners can soften mummified hands by soaking them in chemicals, but in this case the hands were too hard. Zugibe went to New York City's American Museum of Natural History for help. The museum staff allowed him to experiment with different chemicals on pieces of mummies in their collection. After many failed efforts Zugibe finally found a chemical bath that worked. He soaked the corpse's hands in this solution for three days. As he had hoped, the skin softened,

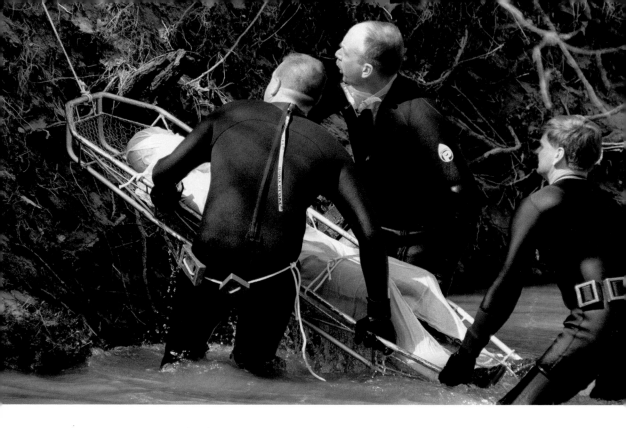

Police divers retrieve the body of a murder victim from a river.

the fingerprints became clear, and Zugibe was able to take fingerprints. With this information detectives were able to discover the woman's identity and eventually catch her murderer.

Pulled from the Water

Identification is only one problem that medical examiners have with decomposing bodies. Sometimes the cause of death can be extremely difficult to determine. Baden tried to discover the cause of death with a partial body found in a lake in New York. The body was a woman's, with neither head nor hands. It was covered in green algae, which are tiny, slimy plants that float in water. Baden scraped off some of the algae and took them to a biologist who examined the samples with his microscope. The biologist found fresh green plants, but he also saw brown plants that had lived on the body the year before. Baden now knew that the body had been in the water at least a year and a half. Next he examined the bones where head and hands should have been attached. He found saw marks on the bones, suggesting homicide. He also examined the bones and the uterus to estimate the woman's age. He determined that the woman was about fifty-five years old.

When the woman's description and possible time of disappearance were given to police, they found a woman who thought the dead body was that of her sister. She even described the last meal she and the woman had shared before the disappearance—fruit and vegetables. Baden had found fruit and vegetables in the corpse's stomach. With Baden's evidence and the sister's identification, police quickly found a suspect in the murder, but they never found out exactly how the woman was killed.

Cause of Death: Unknown

Bodies found in water give up some of their secrets but not all. The bodies of Laci Peterson and her unborn baby, Conner, washed ashore in the San Francisco Bay in April 2003. Medical examiner Brian Peterson (no relation) performed the autopsies on both bodies. They had been in the water for more than four months. Laci's body had no head, was missing both arms and parts of both legs, and had no internal organs except the uterus.

Investigators prepare to transport the body of murder victim Laci Peterson to the morgue for autopsy.

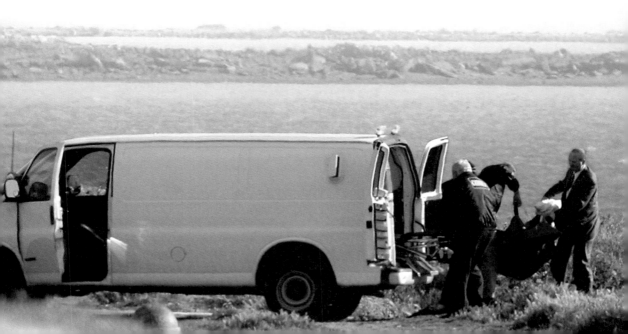

A large tear in the abdominal wall suggested that Conner had floated out of the uterus as his mother's body decomposed.

The medical examiner was able to use DNA testing to identify both bodies. He was able to identify broken ribs on Laci's body and to tell that the baby had been protected in her uterus for a long time. However, he was unable to establish a cause of death for either. The bodies were too decomposed. The manner of death was homicide, but exactly how the two were killed remained unknown, even though Laci's husband was convicted of the murders.

Exhumation

Bodies that have been embalmed and/or buried in coffins do not decompose as quickly as those in water or air. To solve cold cases, bodies are sometimes exhumed, or dug up after burial,

A casket containing the body of a long-dead person is removed from the grave, part of a reinvestigation of an old murder case.

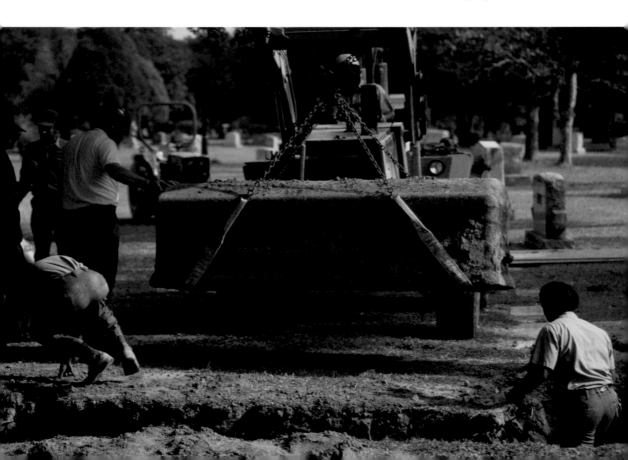

and re-autopsied to search for evidence. If the coffin has re-mained dry, the body may tell a valuable story.

In 1963 Medgar Evers, a civil rights leader, was shot to death in Mississippi. The murderer was suspected but never convicted. Thirty years later, Baden was asked to re-autopsy the exhumed body to help bring Evers's killer to justice. When the coffin was opened, Baden was amazed by the state of the body. He says, "Medgar Evers looked as though he had died only the day before."[51] Baden X-rayed the body and discovered bullet fragments from a bullet that had shattered as it struck a rib. Baden removed and preserved all the fragments. Those fragments matched a gun owned by the suspected murderer. Byron De La Beckwith was convicted of the killing and died in prison in 2001.

The exhumation of Medgar Evers led to a successful autopsy and closed an old murder case. The cause of death was obvious, and the trace evidence was clear and undisturbed. Sometimes, however, even with a medical examiner's best efforts, cause of death remains undetermined. Despite their skills, medical examiners can disagree with one another about an autopsy's meaning or fail to make the body tell the story of its death.

CHAPTER 5

Getting the Story Right

A medical examiner's ultimate objective is to establish details of death so completely that the murderer is identified. "Analyze the evidence to catch the killer. This aim is the Holy Grail of all forensic pathology,"[52] says Zugibe. Forensic pathology is first of all about science, but it is also about putting together the pieces of the story that a body has to tell. When a medical examiner writes the final autopsy report or testifies in court, he or she must give an expert opinion about the meaning of the autopsy story. The accuracy of the ME's opinion depends both on medical skill and the ability to interpret the results. Yet, forensic conclusions are not always as certain as a medical examiner would like them to be. Even the best medical examiners can disagree with one another, make mistakes, or be unable to discover death's complete story.

Not Enough Information

In 1998 twelve-year-old Stephanie Crowe was found stabbed to death in her bedroom. Initially, police investigators believed that the crime was committed by her fourteen-year-old brother and two of his friends. A 6-inch (15.24cm) knife had been found underneath one of the boys' beds. After extensive interrogation two of the boys even confessed to the crime. A year later, however, another person was arrested for the killing. He was a homeless, mentally ill man named Richard Tuite, who had been seen near Stephanie's home. DNA profiling found Stephanie's blood on Tuite's sweatshirt. Lawyers for the boys were sure that their innocence had been established. Lawyers for Tuite argued that the police had mistakenly contaminated Tuite's sweatshirt when they collected it or while testing it.

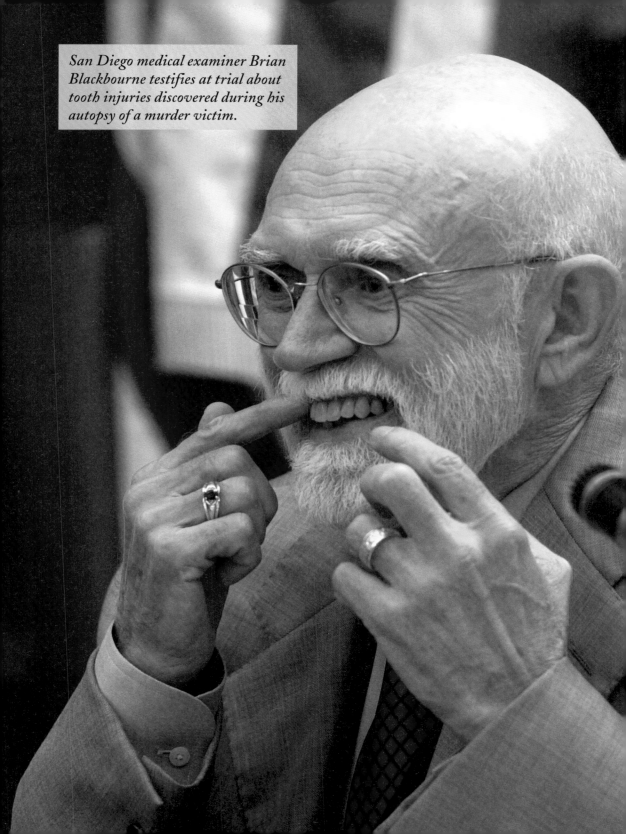

San Diego medical examiner Brian Blackbourne testifies at trial about tooth injuries discovered during his autopsy of a murder victim.

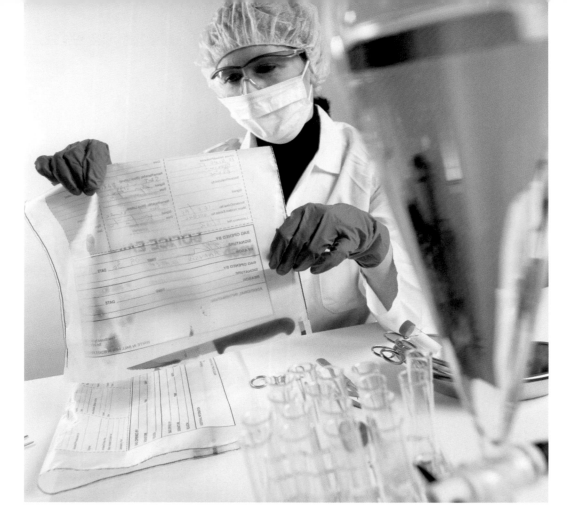

A forensic scientist wearing protective garments to prevent contamination of trace evidence prepares to analyze a crime scene knife for fingerprints, hairs, and blood.

Some police still believed the boys were guilty; others thought Tuite had done the killing. In 2003 Tuite was charged with the murder.

In court San Diego County medical examiner Brian Blackbourne was pressured by both sides for evidence that he could not supply. Blackbourne's autopsy had revealed nine stab wounds, two of which were fatal and caused the girl to bleed to death. He had determined the cause, manner, and mechanism of death, but lawyers and investigators wanted to know more about the knife that had been used. Blackbourne could say that one of the wounds exactly matched a 6-inch (15.24cm) knife, but others could have been made by a larger knife. He could not tell from the autopsy whether or not Tuite was wrongly accused. He could not rule out the knife that belonged to Stephanie's brother. Finally, Blackbourne had to say, "I'm sure there are thousands of knives that could have done this."[53]

Eventually the boys were exonerated, and a jury convicted Tuite of Stephanie's murder. Questions still remained in the minds of the public and some forensic detectives, but they were questions that Blackbourne's autopsy could not answer. An autopsy rarely provides all the evidence needed to catch a killer.

Lost Information

Finding answers is even more difficult when the medical examiner's information is incomplete. A medical examiner cannot interpret evidence that is not there or has been contaminated. If the ME is unable to control the crime scene, for example, evidence and answers may be lost forever.

Lost and contaminated evidence was a major problem when O.J. Simpson's ex-wife Nicole and her friend Ronald Goldman were found stabbed to death outside Nicole's home in 1994. The first police investigators to arrive did not properly protect the crime scene. They walked through blood on a walkway, handled the bodies, and failed to search the house properly for trace evidence. No medical examiner or death investigator was called to the scene until ten hours after the discovery of the bodies. Baden says, "This tragic mistake left unresolved the question of when the victims died."[54] A medical examiner could have checked the bodies for rigor mortis, which indicates time of death most accurately in the first hours of gradual stiffening.

The bloody glove said to belong to the killer of Nicole Brown Simpson and Ronald Goldman lies on the sidewalk at the crime scene.

Then the ME would have checked the crime scene for trace evidence and investigated the house. Baden explains, "The medical examiner would have gone into the residence and looked inside everything—medicine chests, garbage cans, cupboards, the refrigerator—and would have documented what was on the stove and in the sink, in search of anything of medical significance. All this would have been photographed and saved." He adds, "The police are not accustomed to looking at pill bottles, food packages, alcohol bottles, and the like and making the connection to the lives lived by the people who consumed their contents. Medical examiners are."[55]

An investigator for the Boulder, Colorado, County Coroner's Office looks at evidence taken from the scene of JonBenet Ramsey's murder.

In another major error, someone turned Nicole's body over and, in an attempt to be respectful, covered her with a sheet from her house. Police photographs of Nicole's body later showed that the blood of a third party—perhaps her killer—stained her uncut back. When the body was turned over and

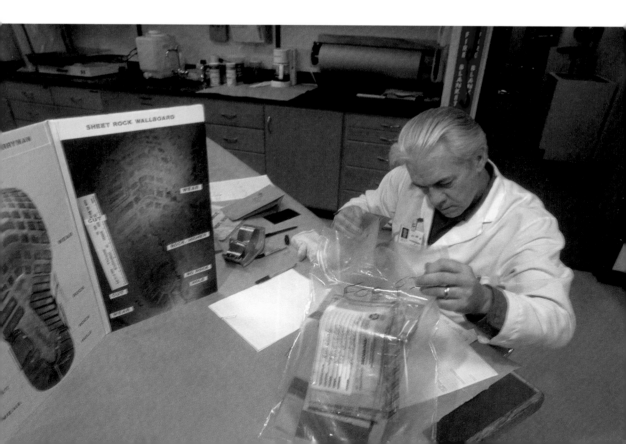

covered, this evidence was lost to the medical examiner forever. The sheet from the house, of course, exchanged trace evidence from the house with the body, making the body useless as a crime scene.

Investigators with bloody shoes also walked from the crime scene to O.J. Simpson's home. Some then returned to the scene of the murders. As Locard's Exchange Principle predicts, they carried trace evidence from one scene to another and contaminated both places. Another police crime scene photo showed a bloody piece of paper beside Nicole's head. It disappeared and was never found. Baden wondered if it was carried away on the shoe of a detective. He says, "I didn't see any evidence planted at the crime scene. No one had to. The police and other visitors tragically and inadvertently brought in and took away trace evidence on their feet, on their clothing, and with their own hands."[56] In part because the medical examiner never took control of the crime scene, no perpetrator was ever convicted for the two murders. O.J. Simpson was tried for the crimes but found not guilty.

A Frustrated Investigation

In another notorious murder case, that of six-year-old JonBenet Ramsey, the county coroner's on-scene investigation was thwarted, too. JonBenet was found murdered in the basement of her parents' home in Boulder, Colorado, on the day after Christmas in 1996. Police tried to protect the scene by letting no one enter the house. Amazingly, when forensic pathologist John Meyer arrived, police would not let him in without a search warrant. Medical examiners do not need search warrants to enter crime scenes. Yet, in a major mistake, Meyer did not gain access to JonBenet's body until six hours after the crime was discovered. He had no way to protect or investigate the crime scene during all that time.

For a television news interview, Zugibe noted another mistake that he believed was made in the medical examiner's investigation. No attempt was made to determine time of death

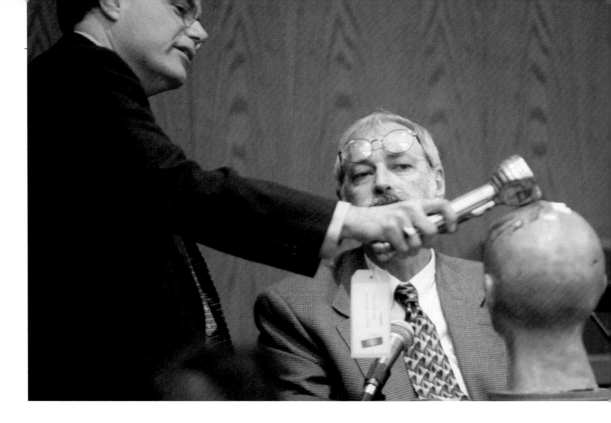

A forensic scientist testifies about his reexamination of old evidence in the 1950s case of the murder of Sam Sheppard's wife.

by checking for body temperature, livor mortis, or rigor mortis. Any information about time of death was lost forever by that omission. The Boulder police disagreed with Zugibe. Officials said that estimates of time of death are inexact and too often inaccurate to be considered important. Zugibe countered that his experience suggested otherwise, especially in the first few hours after death. He said, "As we have seen many times, determining time of death in a homicide is the first and arguably *the* most important job a medical examiner must attempt."[57]

Interpretations in Question

At times medical examiners and police investigators disagree with each other, but medical examiners may disagree with one another, too. Two or more medical examiners may have different opinions about how to interpret autopsy findings. Baden says, "As a medical examiner I know that at any time some other professional may come and review my work. He might be someone come to back me up or someone from the opposite side brought in to review things. . . . Everything we do, in fact, is done so that another person can come in and make an independent assessment, not relying on us."[58] When medical examiners disagree and testify in court, it is the jury that must ultimately decide whom to believe.

In one very old case from the 1950s, for example, two medical experts disagreed about the meaning of blood on a wristwatch. Sam Sheppard had been tried and found guilty of killing his wife in a bloody beating. The only blood found on Sheppard was spattered on his wristwatch. Police said he had cleaned up any other blood before calling them. Sheppard was sent to prison but always claimed he was innocent. After ten years in prison, Sheppard was given a new trial in 1966.

The coroner testified for the prosecution that the way blood was spattered on the watch was consistent with Sheppard being present when his wife was hit. Criminologist Paul Kirk testified for the defense. He said the blood pattern was consistent with smearing of blood from the dead body to Sheppard as Sheppard was

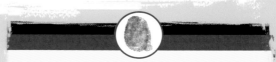

Reading Blood Evidence

Herb MacDonell is known as "the father of blood spatter analysis" in solving crimes. At the Blood Stain Evidence Institute in Corning, New York, MacDonell holds classes and teaches forensic scientists, death investigators, and police detectives to read the story of spilled blood. Using real packages of blood, students come to blood school to learn to understand the pattern in which blood falls, sprays, splatters, and gushes. In one activity, a student takes a mouthful of blood and blows it on different surfaces, including another student. This experiment imitates what would happen if a shooting victim were coughing and dying, and another person ran up to help the victim. Students learn to tell the difference between the splatter of blood from coughing and the back spatter pattern that might occur if a murderer was splashed by blood while shooting someone. The students at the blood school learn how to read any blood pattern that they find in a death investigation from the foremost authority in the world.

checking his wife's pulse when he found her body. "Consistent" is always used by medical examiners to describe their findings and opinions. They know that nothing in their profession is 100 percent certain. The jury heard both opinions, found Sheppard not guilty, and set him free. No one can know for sure which interpretation was correct. The jury had to make the final decision.

Too Many MEs

Three medical examiners investigated the evidence when Ted Binion died in 1998, and all three had different interpretations of the facts. Binion, a drug user and gambler, was found dead on the floor of his Las Vegas home. Eventually, Binion's live-in girlfriend Sandy Murphy and her lover Rick Tabish were accused of murder and brought to trial. Medical examiner Larry Simms did the autopsy and determined that Binion had died of a drug overdose, one too large to be accidental. Simms found the means of death to be drug poisoning and the manner of death to be homicide. Simms testified for the prosecution that someone had given a lethal dose of drugs to Binion.

Baden examined the autopsy evidence and also found the manner of death to be homicide, but for a different reason. He did not believe the toxicology report indicated a lethal amount of drugs. Instead, he thought Binion, a heavy drug user, had taken the drugs himself. However, Baden noted petechial hemorrhages in Binion's eyes that suggested he had been smothered. He also noticed a series of small circular bruises on Binion's chest, as well as other bruises on his lips. Baden testified that someone had smothered Binion by pressing something like a hand over his nose and mouth. When asked to interpret the bruises on Binion's chest, Baden said, "The circular bruises are from shirt buttons."[59] The murderer's buttons had pressed into Binion's chest as he was held down and killed.

Medical examiner Cyril Wecht testified for the defense. He reviewed the autopsy evidence and came to a different conclusion. Wecht testified that Binion's death was a suicide. He said Binion had purposefully taken an overdose of drugs and that he did "not find any evidence to support that contention that he was suffocated."[60] He explained that heavy drug users often have suicidal thoughts.

The evidence was so contradictory that it took hearings, a trial, appeals, and a new trial before the legal system reached

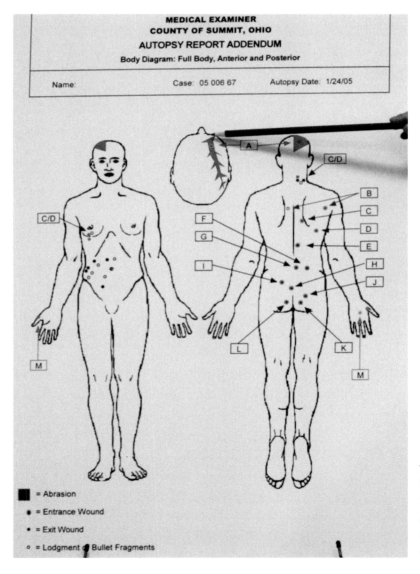

A medical examiner's report usually includes a diagram showing the location of wounds on a victim's body.

A Notorious Method of Murder

Burking is killing by stuffing two fingers in a victim's nostrils to block the airway and clamping the mouth shut with a thumb or elbow. This method of suffocation is named for William Burke, who committed a series of such killings in Edinburgh, Scotland, in 1827 and 1828. Burke and his partner William Hare were paid by a doctor, Robert Knox, to bring him any dead bodies that could be used in anatomy classes. Since they could not find enough bodies dead from natural causes, the two men resorted to murder. There were rumors that Knox taught Burke this method of killing, but Knox's involvement was never proved. The murders created such revulsion in the population when they were discovered that this kind of suffocation has been known as "burking" ever since.

a final conclusion in May 2005. Murphy and Tabish were initially found guilty of murder, but at their new trial the jury set them free. Said one juror, "I think it is really important that if someone is going to say someone's been murdered, you've got to find out how the guy actually died. How do you expect a jury to say murder when you don't really know for sure if it was burking [suffocation] or overdose?"[61] So many conflicting expert opinions about the cause and manner of death were too much for the jury.

A Mistake Corrected

Sometimes conflicting opinions are due to honest mistakes rather than different interpretations of the same facts. When that happens both medical examiners are glad to get the story straight. When Gail Morris was found dead, for example, police believed that she had been beaten to death. She was an alcoholic, found dead in an abandoned car. Police arrested her drinking buddy Leonard Barco for the crime. Barco, who could not remember what he had done, confessed to the murder during interrogation.

Medical examiner Gennaro Braga did Morris's autopsy. He was not a trained forensic pathologist and interpreted the bruises on the body as evidence that Barco's confession was true. He determined that the victim had been beaten and strangled. Barco's lawyer asked Baden to examine the autopsy evidence, and Baden found no evidence of murder. The bruises seemed to be from drunken falls, not a beating. Morris's windpipe and hyoid bone were not fractured. There were no petechial hemorrhages in her eyes. The toxicology report on Morris's blood samples indicated an alcohol level of 0.46—a lethal amount. Baden discovered that Morris had had epileptic seizures as well. Such seizures are worsened by alcohol and could have killed the victim. Baden testified in court that Morris had not been murdered but had died of alcohol poisoning.

When he saw the results of Baden's investigation, Braga apologized to the court. He realized he had made a mistake. He had not read the toxicology report before signing his autopsy findings and was grateful to Baden for catching the error. Barco was released from jail since both medical examiners agreed that the death was an accident.

Limited to One Task

With a complete and careful investigation, medical examiners can often use their science to free the innocent or to identify the guilty. Usually, without disagreement, they can put together the story of a death. At times, however, the best that forensic pathology has to offer is not enough. Zugibe says, "Sometimes forensic science can do nothing to solve a crime. It can only bring a sense of completeness to the events of a death, and to some humble extent, provide a feeling of 'at least we *know*' to those who would otherwise spend the remainder of their lives in a state of constant and painful wondering."[62] This was the

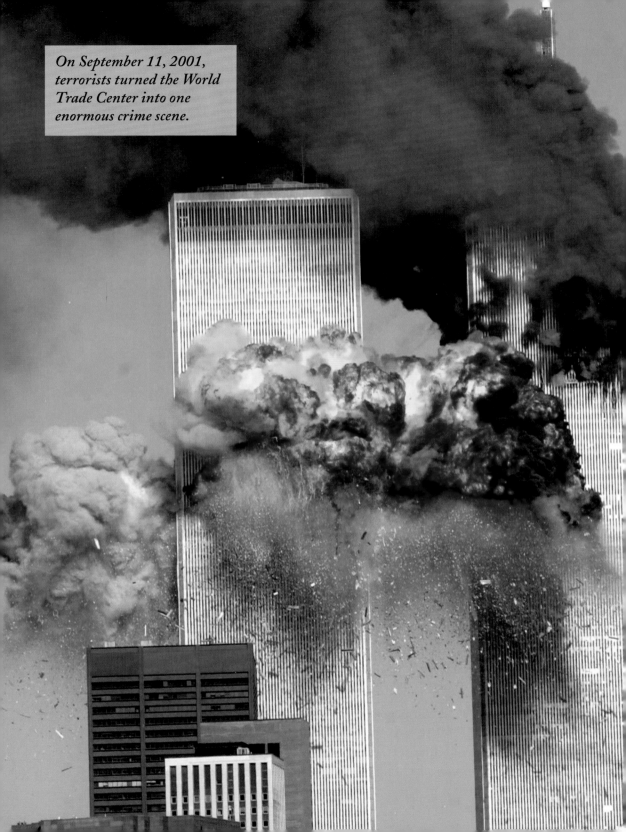

On September 11, 2001, terrorists turned the World Trade Center into one enormous crime scene.

situation on September 11, 2001, when the World Trade Center towers in New York were attacked by terrorists in airplanes. Cause and manner of death were not in question for any of the victims. Time of death was already known. The perpetrators were known. Charles Hirsch, chief medical examiner of New York City, said that his "dialogue with the dead" was limited to one question: "Who are you?"[63]

The World Trade Center was essentially one huge crime scene. Hirsch and six of his staff went to the site immediately after the first plane struck. When the first tower fell, Hirsch was knocked to the ground, cut, bruised, and covered in concrete dust. As he picked himself up, he noticed the fine powder in his pockets. He remembered thinking, "If reinforced concrete was rendered into dust, then it wasn't much of a mystery as to what would happen to people."[64] All Hirsch and his staff could do to help solve the crime was to use all their skills to identify the victims' remains.

Almost twenty thousand body parts were recovered from the crime scene and brought to the medical examiner's office. Hirsch's office and laboratory teams across the country conducted the largest forensic investigation ever to occur in the United States. Most of what the investigators had to work with were bits of badly decomposed tissue and shards of bones containing burned, damaged DNA. Nevertheless, Hirsch and his team members were determined to identify every person they could and return the remains to their loved ones. Using DNA profiling, they spent years matching victim remains to DNA samples from hairbrushes, toothbrushes, pillowcases, and razors brought in by relatives of the victims. Their goal was to help the living and honor the dead by giving an identity to each and every piece of human remains.

Stalled, but Not Defeated

More than half the World Trade Center victims have been identified, but no trace has been found of the remains of more than eleven hundred victims. The science of forensic pathology is not advanced enough to make accurate matches with all the bits of broken-down DNA. On February 23, 2005, the medical examiner's office announced that efforts to identify victims had reached their limits. A spokesperson for the medical examiner's office, however, said, "This is a pause—we've exhausted the limits of the technology as it exists today. But the doctors have promised—*promised*—that we will never say 'case closed.'"[65]

Today, Hirsch's office is carefully preserving and storing all the unidentified body parts that could not be returned to their families for burial. The hope is that forensic pathologists in

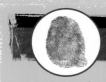

DNA Test Pioneers

At the World Trade Center, DNA was degraded because of extremely hot fires that burned for weeks, moisture that encouraged decay, and bacteria that speeded up decomposition. The cell walls and nuclei of victims' remains broke down. The strings of base pairs of the DNA ladder fell apart. The base pair strands that were left were so small that they could not be tested for matches. Sometimes only sixty to eighty base pairs were found in a sample, as opposed to the hundreds or thousands that are available for testing in fresh DNA. Standard DNA profiling techniques were useless for making matches. Efforts to develop a DNA profile with this degraded DNA usually came back from the lab marked "incomplete" or "negative."

The New York medical examiner's office began using a new scientific technique called SNPS (single nucleotide polymorphisms) to search for the smallest variations in their samples. SNPS testing is not as reliable as standard tests. The chance of a match being incorrect is only about one in forty-six hundred instead of one in billions. Nevertheless, many scientists worked to validate the technique as an identification method, and a few remains were identified with this SNPS process.

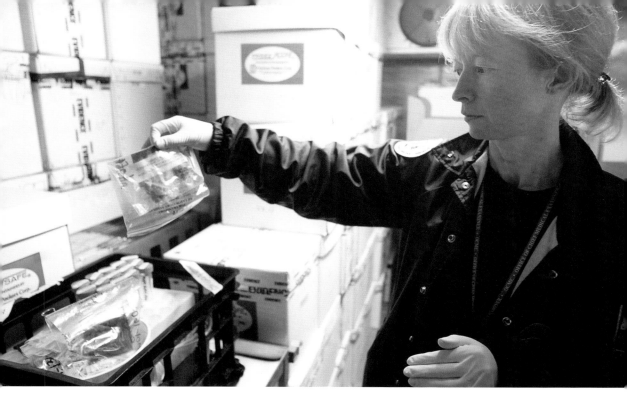

the future will develop new technology that will allow these remains to be identified. Says Hirsch, "It's important to people and we're here to serve people. If a government can't do that, what good is it?"[66]

Medical examiners work with the dead, but their ultimate goal is to help society and to bring comfort and answers to the living who have lost loved ones. Their efforts have failed with many 9/11 victims, but they vow never to give up. Medical examiners often quote an inscription on the wall in the New York City Office of the Chief Medical Examiner. It expresses their belief in the purpose of their profession: "Let conversation cease. Let laughter flee. This is the place where death delights to help the living."[67]

A forensic scientist in New York City holds samples of unidentified human remains recovered from the ruins of the World Trade Center.

Notes

Introduction

1. Thomas T. Noguchi with Joseph DiMona, *Coroner*. Boston: G.K. Hall, 1983, pp. 3–4.

Chapter 1: At the Death Scene

2. Frederick Zugibe and David L. Carroll, *Dissecting Death*. New York: Broadway Books, 2005, p. 153.

3. Zugibe and Carroll, *Dissecting Death*, p. 39.

4. Zugibe and Carroll, *Dissecting Death*, p. 153.

5. Michael M. Baden and Marion Roach, *Dead Reckoning*. New York: Simon and Schuster, 2001, p. 149.

6. Baden and Roach, *Dead Reckoning*, p. 21.

7. Baden and Roach, *Dead Reckoning*, pp. 20–21, 140.

8. Noguchi, *Coroner*, p. 304.

9. Noguchi, *Coroner*, pp. 257–58.

10. Zugibe and Carroll, *Dissecting Death*, p. 44.

11. Quoted in Kelly M. Pyrek, "As Death Investigators, Nurses Pick Up on Crime-Scene Subtleties," *Forensic Nurse*. www.forensicnursemag.com/articles/ 311feat1.html.

12. Zugibe and Carroll, *Dissecting Death*, p. 157.

13. Baden and Roach, *Dead Reckoning*, pp. 17, 22.

14. Baden and Roach, *Dead Reckoning*, p. 20.

Chapter 2: Autopsy

15. Jay Dix and Robert Calaluce, *Guide to Forensic Pathology*. Boca Raton, FL: CRC, 1998, pp. 30, 14.

16. Baden and Roach, *Dead Reckoning*, p. 14.

17. Baden and Roach, *Dead Reckoning*, p. 20.

18. Quoted in Zugibe and Carroll, *Dissecting Death*, p. 181.

19. Zugibe and Carroll, *Dissecting Death*, p. 34.

20. Dix and Calaluce, *Guide to Forensic Pathology*, p. 75.

21. Noguchi, *Coroner*, p. 260.

22. Zugibe and Carroll, *Dissecting Death*, p. 199.

23. Dix and Calaluce, *Guide to Forensic Pathology*, pp. 159–60.

24. Zugibe, *Dissecting Deth*, pp. 140–41.

25. Michael M. Baden with Judith Adler Hennessee, *Unnatural Death: Confessions of a Medical Examiner.* New York: Random House, 1989, p. 98.

26. Baden, *Unnatural Death*, p. 103.

27. Baden and Roach, *Dead Reckoning*, p. 111.

28. Dix and Calaluce, *Guide to Forensic Pathology*, p. 181.

Chapter 3: Poison, Blood, and DNA

29. Quoted in Raymond Hardie, "One in a Trillion: On the Job: David Fisher, '97," *UCSD Alumni Magazine*, vol. 1 no. 3, September 2004. http://alumni.ucsd.edu/magazine/vol1no3/features/trillion.htm.

30. D.P. Lyle, *Forensics for Dummies.* Hoboken, NJ: Wiley, 2004, p. 209.

31. Lyle, *Forensics for Dummies*, p. 267.

32. Katherine Ramsland, "Modern Detection Methods," Court TV's Crime Library. www.crimelibrary.com/criminal_mind/forensics/toxicology/l0.html?sect=21.

33. Lyle, *Forensics for Dummies*, p. 244.

34. Noguchi, *Coroner*, pp. 267–68.

35. Quoted in Seamus McGraw, "Perfect Poison," in *Death in the Family: The Rose Petal Murder*, Court TV's Crime Library. www.crimelibrary.com/notorious%5Fmurders/family/kristen%5Frossum.

36. Zugibe and Carroll, *Dissecting Death*, p. 26.

37. Quoted in Emanuella Grinberg, "Teen's Family Asks Judge to Keep Her in Prison for Life," Court TV. www.courttv.com/trials/johnson/062905_sentence_ctv.html.

38. Quoted in *CBS News*, "Who Murdered the Rock Star?"*48 Hours,* January 8, 2005. www.cbsnews.com/stories/2004/05/14/48hours/main617479.shtml.

39. Quoted in *CBS News*, "Who Murdered the Rock Star?"

40. Quoted in *CBS News*, "Who Murdered the Rock Star?"

Chapter 4: Decomposition

41. Luv Sharma et al., "Second Autopsy— a Bane or a Boon!" *Anil Aggrawal's Internet Journal of Forensic Medicine and Toxicology*, vol.4, no. 2, July/December/2003.www.geradts.com/anil/ij/vol_004_no_002/papers/paper004.html.

42. Zugibe and Carroll, *Dissecting Death*, pp. 89–90.

43. M. Lee Goff, *A Fly for the Prosecution.* Cambridge, MA: Harvard University Press, 2000, p. 45.

44. Zugibe and Carroll, *Dissecting Death*, p. 91.

45. Goff, *A Fly for the Prosecution*, p. 49.

46. Zugibe and Carroll, *Dissecting Death*, p. 92.

47. Goff, *A Fly for the Prosecution*, p. 7.

48. Baden and Roach, *Dead Reckoning*, p. 207.

49. Baden and Roach, *Dead Reckoning*, p. 115.

50. Zugib and Carroll, *Dissecting Death*, p. 15.

51. Baden and Roach, *Dead Reckoning*, p. 194.

Chapter 5: Getting the Story Right

52. Zugibe and Carroll, *Dissecting Death*, p. 213.

53. Quoted in John Springer, "At Hearing, A Question: Which Knife Was Used to Kill Stephanie Crowe?" CourtTV.com. www.courttv.com/trials/tuite/020603_ctv.html.

54. Baden and Roach, *Dead Reckoning*, p. 150.

55. Baden and Roach, *Dead Reckoning* p. 151.

56. Baden and Roach, *Dead Reckoning*, p. 148.

57. Zugibe and Carroll, *Dissecting Death*, p. 230.

58. Baden and Roach, *Dead Reckoning*, p. 74.

59. Baden and Roach, *Dead Reckoning*, p. 88.

60. Quoted in Baden and Roach, *Dead Reckoning*, pp. 89–90.

61. Quoted in Glenn Puit, "Murder Trial of Murphy, Tabish: Binion Jurors Explain Vote to Acquit," *Las Vegas Review_Journal*, May 8, 2005. www.reviewjournal.com/lvrj-home/2005/Mav-08-Sun-2005/news/26469881.html.

62. Zugibe and Carroll, *Dissecting Death*, p. 225.

63. Quoted in Dan Barry, "At Morgue, Ceaselessly Sifting 9/11 Traces," *9/11 Stories and Articles*, July 17, 2002. www.werismyki.com/articles/ceaselessly_sifting.html.

64. Quoted in Barry, "At Morgue, Ceaselessly Sifting 9/11 Traces."

65. Quoted in Michael Powell, "Identification of 9/11 Victims Reaches Limits of Technology," *Washington Post.com*, February, 24, 2005, p. A03. www.washingtonpost.com/wp-dyn/articles/A47866-2005Feb23.html.

66. Quoted in Barry, "At Morgue, Ceaselessly Sifting 9/11 Traces."

67. Quoted in Baden, *Unnatural Death*, p. 31.

For Further Reading

Books

Ron Fridell, *Solving Crimes: Pioneers of Forensic Science*. Danbury, CT: Franklin Watts, Grolier, 2000. Explore the lives of six people who used forensic science to change the way crime is investigated. Read the story of Edmund Locard and learn about Alec Jeffreys's first efforts at DNA profiling.

Barbara B. Rollins and Michael Dahl, *Blood Evidence*. Mankato, MN: Capstone, 2004. This easy-to-read book describes using blood evidence to solve crimes, complete with gruesome pictures.

Pam Walker and Elaine Wood, *Crime Scene Investigations: Real Life Science Labs for Grades 6–12*. San Francisco: Jossey-Bass, 2002. Solve crimes with these experiments by identifying toolmarks, examining blood drops, and protecting the crime scene.

Internet Sources

Ann Meeker-O'Connell, "How DNA Evidence Works," *HowStuffWorks*. www. howstuffworks.com/dna-evidence.htm. Explore the technology of DNA profiling.

Ed Uthman, "Autopsy Tools." http://web2. iadfw.net/uthman/autopsy_tools.html. This page shows the photos and names of many of the tools used in an autopsy.

Robert Valdes, "How Autopsies Work." *HowStuffWorks*. http://health.howstuff works.com/autopsy.htm. Follow the steps of a medical examiner as he performs an autopsy, and learn some odd facts about the chances of dying in very unusual ways. There are plenty of photographs, but none are of bodies.

Web Site

Virtual Tour: State of Tennessee Center for Forensic Medicine (www.forensic med.com/virtual_tour.htm). Take a virtual tour of the forensic center, including the medical examiner's main autopsy room.

Works Consulted

Books

Michael M. Baden with Judith Adler Hennessee, *Unnatural Death: Confessions of a Medical Examiner*. New York: Random House, 1989. Baden describes his professional life as a New York medical examiner and comments on illustrative forensic cases.

Michael M. Baden and Marion Roach, *Dead Reckoning*. New York: Simon and Schuster, 2001. Baden discusses many of the well-known cases with which he has been involved and explains the science of forensic pathology.

Tony Blanche and Brad Schreiber, *Death in Paradise*. Los Angeles: GPG, 1998. A popularized look at the history of the coroner in Los Angeles County.

Catherine Crier, *A Deadly Game*. New York: HarperCollins, 2005. The author presents a detailed examination of the Scott Peterson murder trial.

Jay Dix and Robert Calaluce, *Guide to Forensic Pathology*. Boca Raton, FL: CRC, 1998. The authors provide a scholarly examination of forensic pathology for death investigators and medical students.

M. Lee Goff, *A Fly for the Prosecution*. Cambridge, MA: Harvard University Press, 2000. This lively account of a forensic entomologist's career describes not only his research and case studies, but also the struggle for professional recognition.

D.P. Lyle, *Forensics for Dummies*. Hoboken, NJ: Wiley, 2004. This sometimes humorous overview of the field of forensic science covers every aspect of an investigation and includes numerous examples.

Thomas T. Noguchi with Joseph DiMona, *Coroner*. Boston, MA: G.K. Hall, 1983. Noguchi describes his life as the chief medical examiner for Los Angeles County, when he was known as the "coroner to the stars."

Lawrence Schiller and James Willwerth, *American Tragedy: The Uncensored Story of the Simpson Defense*. New York: Random House, 1996. A detailed account of the people involved in and events before and during the O.J. Simpson murder trial.

Frederick Zugibe and David L. Carroll, *Dissecting Death*. New York: Broadway Books, 2005. Zugibe discusses the adventures of a New York medical examiner and provides readable explanations of his science.

Internet Sources

Dan Barry, "At Morgue, Ceaselessly Sifting 9/11 Traces", *9/11 Stories and Articles*, July 17, 2002. www.werismyki.com/articles/ceaselessly-sifting.html.

Jon Callas, "Limits of DNA Research Pushed to Identify the Dead of Sept. 11," *New York Times*, April 22, 2002; repr. at Eristocracy: The Mail Archive. www.mail-archive.com/eristocracy@merrymeet.com/msg00031.html.

CBS News, "Who Murdered the Rock Star?" *48 Hours,* January 8, 2005. www.cbsnews.com/stories/2004/05/14/48hours/main617479.shtml.

Christine Clarridge, "Zapata's Killer Gets 36 Years," *Seattle Times,* May 1, 2004. http://seattletimes.nwsource.com/html/localnews/2001917473_zapata01m.html.

Thomas Curran, preparer, *Forensic DNA Analysis: Technology and Application*: Library of Parliament, September 1997 [Canada]. http://www.parl.gc.ca/information/library/PRBpubs/bp443-e.htm.

Lynne Duke, "Doctor Who: Biologist Bob Shaler Hunts for Names Amid the Remains of 9/11," *Washington Post.com,* September 7, 2003. http:// ocean.otr.usm.edu/~ddavies/courses/doctorwho.html.

Marcella Fierro, "Medical Examiners Aid Both Living, Dead," *Richmond Times-Dispatch,* February 8, 2004; repr. Virginia Institute of Forensic Science and Medicine: News. www.vifsm.org/news/2004/0224medical_examiner_oped.htm.

Mark Gribben, "Michael Fletcher: A Simple Case of Murder," *Court TV's Crime Library.* www.crimelibrary.com/notorious_murders/family/fletcher/1.html.

Emanuella Grinberg, "Teen's Family Asks Judge to Keep Her in Prison for Life," *Court TV.* www.courttv.com/trials/johnson/062905_sentence_ctv.html.

Raymond Hardie, "One in a Trillion: On the Job: David Fisher, '97," *UCSD Alumni Magazine,* vol. 1, no. 3, September 2004. http://alumni.ucsd.edu/magazine/vol1no.3/features/trillion.htm.

HBO, "Ask Dr. Baden," *Autopsy.* www.hbo.com/autopsy/baden/qa_2.html.

King County Medical Examiner's Office 2003 Annual Report. http://www.metrokc.gov/health/examiner/2003report/Index.htm.

Eric Lipton, "At Limits of Science, 9/11 ID Effort Comes to End," *New York Times,* July 10, 2005. www.rinf.com/news/ap-05/04.html.

Seamus McGraw, *Death in the Family: The Rose Petal Murder, Court TV's Crime Library.* www.crimelibrary.com/notorious%5Fmurders/family/kristen%5Frossum.

Martha T. Moore, "NYC's Work to ID 9/11 Victims Ends—For Now", *USA Today,* February 23, 2005. www.usatoday.com/news/sept11/2005-02-23-sept11-ids_x.htm.

Steve Moriarty, "The Trial," The Gits.Com. http://www.thegits.com/miatrial.html.

Patrice O'Shaughnessy, "More Than Half of Victims IDd," *New York Daily News*, September 11, 2002. www.nydailynews. com/news/local/story/17949p-17009c.html.

Michael Powell, "Identification of 9/11 Victims Reaches Limits of Technology," *Washington Post.com*, February 24, 2005. www.washingtonpost.com/wp-dyn/ar ticles/A47866-2005Feb23.html.

Glenn Puit, "Murder Trial of Murphy, Tabish: Binion Jurors Explain Vote to Acquit," *Las Vegas Review-Journal*, May 8, 2005. www.reviewjournal.com/lvrj_ home/2005/May-08-Sun-2005/ news/26469881.html.

Kelly M. Pyrek, "As Death Investigators, Nurses Pick Up on Crime-Scene Subtleties," *Forensic Nurse*. www.foren sicnursemag.com/articles/311feat1.html.

Katherine Ramsland, "Modern Detection Methods," *Court TV's Crime Library*. www.crimelibrary.com/criminal_mind/f orensics/toxicology/10.html?sect=21.

Donald E. Riley, "DNA Testing: An Introduction for Non-Scientists: An Illustrated Explanation," *Scientific Testimony: An Online Journal*, April 6, 2005, www.scientific.org/tutorials/articles/riley /riley.html.

Luv Sharma et al., "Second Autopsy—a Bane or a Boon!" *Anil Aggrawal's Internet Journal of Forensic Medicine and Toxicology*, vol.4, no. 2, July/December 2003. www.geradts.com/anil/ij/vol_004_ no_002/papers/paper004.html.

John Springer, "At Hearing, A Question: Which Knife Was Used to Kill Stephanie Crowe?" *Court TV.com*. www. courttv.com/trials/tuite/020603_ctv.html.

Index

Picture Credits

Cover: © Julie Plasencial/San Francisco Chronicle/CORBIS (main image)
AFP/Getty Images, 12
AP/Wide World Photos, 16, 27, 50, 58, 62, 66, 72, 73, 79, 82, 85
Maury Aaseng, 14, 20, 31, 35, 39, 40
© Ashley Cooper/CORBIS, 11
© Custom Medical Stock Photo, Inc., 7, 31, 40, 41
© Roger Eritja/Alamy, 68
© Maurio Fermariello/Photo Researchers, Inc., 46
© Danny Gawlowski/Dallas Morning News/CORBIS, 64
Getty Images, 88, 91
© Pascal Goetgheluck/Photo Researchers, Inc., 23
© Philip Gould/CORBIS, 74
© James Holmes/Thomson Laboratories/Photo Researchers, Inc., 47
© Mikael Karlsson/Alamy, 51
Axel Koester/CORBIS, 80
© P. Motta/Photo Researchers, Inc., 46
© Najlah/CORBIS, 9
© Gabe Palmer/CORBIS, 45
© David Parker/ Photo Reserachers, Inc., 54
© PASIEKA/Photo Researchers, Inc., 53
© Plain Picture GmbH & Co. KG/Alamy, 19
© Julie Plasencia/San Francisco Chronicle/CORBIS, 8
Reuters/Getty Images, 77
© Alexander Ruesche/EPA/Landov, 24
© Science Source/Photo Researchers, Inc., 29
© Dr. Jurgen Scriba/Photo Researchers, Inc., 52
© Shepard Sherbell/CORBIS, 28, 37
© SNL/DOE/Photo Researchers, Inc., 36
© Volker Steger/Photo Researchers, Inc., 69, 70
© TEK Image/Photo Researchers, Inc., 78

About the Author

Toney Allman holds degrees from Ohio State University and the University of Hawaii. She currently lives in Virginia where she writes nonfiction books for students.